The Truth About Chronic Pain

The Truth About Chronic Pain

*Patients and Professionals
on How to Face It,
Understand It,
Overcome It*

ARTHUR ROSENFELD

BASIC
BOOKS

A Member of the Perseus Books Group

Published by Basic Books,
A Member of the Perseus Books Group

Designed by Brent Wilcox

Library of Congress Cataloging-in-Publication Data
Rosenfeld, Arthur.
   The truth about chronic pain : patients and professionals on how to face it, understand it, overcome it / Arthur Rosenfeld.
      p.   cm.
   ISBN 0-465-07138-4 (hardcover)
   1. Chronic pain.   2. Chronic pain—Patients—Interviews.
[DNLM: 1. Chronic Disease—Interview. 2. Pain—Interview. WL 704
R813t 2003] I. Title.
   RB127 .R664   2003
   616'.0472—dc21

2002151003

03 04 05 / 10 9 8 7 6 5 4 3 2 1

For my father

The quality of mercy is not strain'd,
It droppeth as the gentle rain from heaven
Upon the place beneath: it is twice blest;
It blesseth him that gives and him that takes:
'Tis mightiest in the mightiest: it becomes
The throned monarch better than his crown;
His sceptre shows the force of temporal power,
The attribute to awe and majesty,
Wherein doth sit the dread and fear of kings;
But mercy is above this sceptred sway;
It is enthroned in the hearts of kings,
It is an attribute to God himself;
And earthly power doth then show likest God's
When mercy seasons justice.

THE MERCHANT OF VENICE, ACT 4, SCENE 1

WILLIAM SHAKESPEARE

Contents

Acknowledgments

First and foremost I am grateful to the pain patients interviewed here. Thank you for opening your homes and your hearts to a complete stranger, and for sharing details that were sometimes wrenching, often inspirational, and always intimate.

A bow also goes to the caregivers who gave their honest, considered, and sometimes risky testimony in the pages that follow. Thank you for your candor and your bravery and your passionate devotion to those in pain.

The thinkers and commentators who helped me make sense of the senseless, who dispensed with political correctness and doublespeak to render unerring opinions about our prides and prejudices inside a system that desperately needs fixing deserve kudos as well. Thank you all for taking time from your busy lives to help me ponder the question of why we suffer when we need not.

A huge debt goes to my friends at Purdue Pharma, L.P., without whose unconditional grant this book would not have been possible. Thank you for trusting my instincts, and for making your support of this project completely free of any judgment or bias.

Without my agent, Jack Scovil, this book would not have found the marvelous home it did. Thank you, Jack, for your patience and perseverance. Thank you also to my editor, Jo Ann Miller, at Basic Books, and to her assistant, Candace Taylor, without whom everything would have gotten lost in the shuffle. Thanks to Richard Fumosa for copyediting above and beyond the call of duty.

Thanks also go to my dear friend and teacher Mitch Cantor, who helped me when metaphysics got the better of me, and my friend and teacher Master Gaofei Yan, who literally took me by the shoulders and set me on the path. Last, but not least, thanks to my father, Dr. Isadore Rosenfeld, for his wise and important introduction to this book and to life itself. I love you, Dad.

Foreword

To feel pain is "unhealthy"; to endure it is unnecessary. Hurt is your body's signal that something is awry and needs correcting. When the cause is obvious—a broken bone or an injury—the doctor fixes it and prescribes the necessary medication to make you comfortable. No questions are asked; no guilt or hesitation on anyone's part.

This fascinating book deals with a totally different scenario: the critically important and widespread problem of how doctors and patients react when the reason for the pain is clear but the pain cannot be cured. Because of societal attitudes, millions continue to suffer unnecessarily, day in, day out, from incurable cancers, chronic diseases such as crippling arthritis, and a host of neurological disorders that plague our aging population. The incidence of these "degenerative" diseases is increasing as Americans grow older, and for many, life is full of pain.

It would seem obvious that pain should be relieved whenever possible: Life should be made bearable for those incurably afflicted, especially since there are so many effective ways to do so. Why deny anyone the relief they crave? It should not be an issue of contention, but it is. For there exists in our society a complex interplay of ethics, mores, religious beliefs, dogma, cultural attitudes, all of which arrive at the conclusion, by different routes, that "coping" with pain is, for whatever reason, more "noble" than eliminating it. This attitude, brilliantly investigated in this volume, is embraced not only by many caregivers who withhold the necessary relief, but also by the victims, who feel guilty, weak, and inadequate for requesting it. Their plight is made worse by the fact that in addition to being unable to cure the cause of their pain, medical science can prolong their lives, thus prolonging their misery.

Some of the naysayers among the philosophers, ethicists, physicians and others with whom the author has discussed the question of pain perception and its control invoke the specter of habituation and addiction to justify their stance, even though there is no compelling or convincing scientific basis for this fear. Effects from modern pain medication taken as prescribed—even habituation—are preferable to most of us than unrelenting pain.

The conversations in this book allow us to assess the morality of withholding pain relief in the light of medical progress. It is a breath of fresh air to doctors such as me who have wrestled with our consciences as we attempt to be compassionate to those in distress. It also provides the victims who suffer in silence with the support they may need to reconsider their reticence to receive relief. Although the author explores many sides of the issue, I am certain that he shares my attitudes. They are not only a matter of logic, but as far as he and I are concerned, of genetics as well.

—Isadore Rosenfeld, M.D.

Rossi Distinguished Professor of Clinical Medicine,
   Weill Cornell Medical College
Past president, New York County Medical Society
Health editor, Parade *magazine*

Introduction

There is a saying among motorcycle aficionados that there are three kinds of bike riders: those who have been down, those who are going down, and those who are going down again. Pain and loss, if not agony and death, are inevitable consequences of perching atop two small patches of rubber at high speed, yet thousands of motorcyclists rack up millions of miles every year. If you ask a biker about the trauma he is someday likely to face, he will probably tell you that pain is a part of life, and, that because there is no getting away from it, he might as well enjoy himself until it arrives. Riding a motorcycle may be stacking the odds, but the fact remains that all that differentiates a healthy, pain-free person from a person in chronic pain is age, exposure to a toxin, a pathogen, an act of terror, or, as in Greek tragedies and the aboriginal world, the venom-filled fangs of a snake in the grass.

If pleasure and pain are the twin poles of human experience, and if, as many behaviorists argue, we are driven toward pleasure and away from pain, we ought to have the right to live according to this biological imperative and be as pain free as nature intended. Yet while food stamps assure our right to eat and homeless shelters assure our right to a roof over our heads, nothing in the United States today certifies for us the right to live free from controllable chronic pain. Indeed, chronic pain has reached epidemic proportions in our country: estimates range from 25 million sufferers to 75 million. Unlike the acute pain of a motorcycle accident, or the pain that comes from cancer or AIDS, much chronic pain derives from conditions that are less dramatic, less familiar, and less well understood. Chronic pain may show with a grimace, a cane, a bottle of pills, a short temper, or, in the case of the devout Stoic, it may not show at all. Whatever the exterior landscape reveals, however, the interior landscape of the chronic pain sufferer is barren of self-confidence, enthusiasm, relationships, personality, identity, and ultimately the tiniest shred of joy.

As you read this, you can be certain that someone in your own personal universe is in chronic pain. It may be someone whose life only grazes your own, or it may be someone who shares your standbrush. The cause may be trauma, cancer, diabetes, an autoimmune or inflammatory condition, or one of myriad degenerative diseases of aging, but the stunning fact is that even though most of this pain can be eliminated or greatly reduced, it is not. Despite the fact that we live in the most affluent and technologically advanced nation in the history of the world, millions of people continue to suffer for no good reason at all.

Although chronic pain has not thus far invaded my body, it has pried its way into my soul. Before devoting myself to writing full-time in 1990, I worked for a company that manufactured a line of medications for moderate to severe chronic pain. In that capacity, I became aware that for thousands of people, physical pain careens out of control every day despite the fact that there are techniques and substances to control it. I saw videos, heard testimonials, and encountered patients whose stories were heartbreaking, and I quickly learned that the problem was far more complex than I could have possibly imagined. Some insurance companies put a cap on how much pain medication they pay for. Some people in pain were simply not believed because the source of their pain did not show up on any tests. I found that an inappropriate fear of addiction to opioid analgesics—morphine, codeine, their variants and derivatives—led many patients not to ask for adequate relief until their pain was utterly intolerable. I also discovered, to my dismay, that physicians were often reluctant to prescribe adequate dosages of these medications for fear of turning their patients into drug abusers, despite strong evidence that this was an unlikely eventuality.

Realizing that at least part of the solution was education, I helped launch a successful Internet, print, and video program to educate both physicians and patients about chronic pain. Although this project was gratifying, the ongoing suffering of pain patients weighed heavily on me, all the more so because in those days I went home each night to a wife who had been the victim of a terrible car accident when we had been married for only six months. The severity of her problems, from brain damage to musculoskeletal injuries, kept her in constant distress while simultaneously depriving me of a respite from the draining topic of my work.

At the same time, my uncle, Arthur Master, was slowly dying of metastatic disease. The spread of his cancer proceeded relentlessly during the years I was professionally engaged in the world of chronic pain management. I saw him suffer unimaginable agony when relief was only a small pill away, and I could not understand why that relief was withheld. As he was obviously not going to leave the hospital, the pain of his condition far outweighed any concerns about addiction, and worries about such side effects as respiratory depression or constipation were also misplaced, as a compassionate death would have been the best thing anyone could have wished for him. I became convinced that the best measure of a society is not, as has been suggested, to be found in the way it treats its prisoners, but in the way it cares for its citizens in pain.

The atrocities of inadequate pain management are not trumpeted over the nightly news, even though they transpire right here in our own backyard. This tragedy represents a quiet but intolerable epidemic, all the more devastating because it speaks to values we don't usually discuss, and reflects deeply held prejudices and presumptions as unjust as any and uglier than most. How can we ignore the chronic suffering in our midst? Why are many doctors more willing to give a shot for the flu than a pill for pain? Why are so many of us afraid to ask for relief? Why is our disdain for addiction to narcotics greater than our intolerance of people living and dying in needless agony? What is the root of our uneasiness around suffering?

We have allowed the political and economic aspects of managing pain, the politics of a failed drug war, the suspect motives of insurers and the unchecked greed of some health care professionals to obscure the fact that chronic pain can and will strike anyone, anywhere, anytime. Chaotic, organic, and devastating, chronic pain is a pervasive, nearly universal condition that knows no socioeconomic, racial, or educational boundary.

As I researched the issue, it became clear to me that I could be of greatest service by providing a forum for the views of others rather than by writing a book stating my own views. *The Truth About Chronic Pain* is, therefore, a series of interviews, or, better, a collection of conversations. I selected the people who speak here by tapping sources as diverse as former schoolmates, corporate contacts, and advocacy groups: because the subject can be very personal and sensitive, I ranged across the country for eighteen months to have those conversations face-to-face. Chronic pain sufferers hold forth in the pages that follow, but so do medical pioneers, primary care physicians, educators, legislators, enforcers, clergy, and even a sports hero fallen from grace.

Other books about pain fall either within the category of clinical manuals for the health care professional, self-help books for those suffering pain, or treatises for the academic reader. Although some are rich sources of technical, medical, scientific and cultural information, they lack the single thing they should display in greatest abundance: overarching human warmth and compassion. The subject of chronic pain is, after all, far less about nerve cells and neurotransmitters than it is about the misery of having a nightmare from which there is no awakening. Philosophical abstractions, scientific journeying, and political maneuvering obscure the bristling immediacy and power of needless personal suffering.

Although I strove for a nonjudgmental tone in my questions, I am certain that at times moral outrage and sadness overtook me and my feelings show through. Indeed, no objective arguments can reveal as much about our trials and our misapprehensions, our fears, our systematic failings, and our personal triumphs, as do the passionate, and highly subjective, voices between the covers of this book. *The Truth About Chronic Pain* is neither an exhaustive work of scholarship nor a medical treatise. Rather, it is an exploration of the human dimension of one of the most profound issues that confront us today, an expedition that strikes out, equipped with a high-powered lantern, in search of some of our most deeply buried and closely held secrets.

PART ONE

Patients in Pain

WHILE I WAS WRITING THIS BOOK, PEOPLE OFTEN asked me whether the topic was physical pain or emotional pain. This distinction is, of course, an arbitrary and intellectual one. Severe chronic pain is a state of bondage so total and so hard for nonsufferers to imagine that they simply cannot understand why those in pain would sometimes rather die than continue living without relief. We have no reference point to someone else's pain, but the chronic pain patient's reference point is his suffering. The average American is afflicted with high-level suffering as many as sixty days per year, and yet more than one out of four who suffer wait at least six months before going to a doctor. Young people are more likely to place a positive spin on their pain—what doesn't kill me makes me stronger—seeing it as a useful experience, a tool for growth. Older people do this less often, perhaps because they've endured a lot already and feel that enough is enough. Sensing that they are alone, sensing that the rest of us tend to judge them unfairly or unkindly, pain patients crave validation nearly as keenly as they crave physical release. Some people are so frustrated by the way health care professionals and family and friends treat them that they actually crave a dire diagnosis rather than a nonspecific one.

They'd rather be in grave trouble than be scorned or disbelieved. Words hold their own brand of malignancy, and can hurt nearly as much as a tumor.

Even the deeply religious find it hard to make sense of chronic pain—Why is God doing this to me?—and their bewilderment often leads to despair. Anxiety and depression are planets in orbit about the dark sun of pain. More and more doctors are adding antidepressants to pain control regimens, finding that the medications act not only to elevate mood but also to render the patient measurably more insensate. Claiming that proper pain treatment requires special knowledge, our medical system tends to give control of relief to the doctor, not the patient. This despite the fact that patients handed the reins of their own medication using the devices of Patient-Controlled Analgesia (PCA) are shown to use less medication than patients who are not given control. Lack of control leads to anxiety, which may be medicated with antianxiety drugs known as anxiolytics. In many chronic pain situations, the doctors are men and the patients are women, a situation that adds to the risk of judgment and imprecation. Lacking power, chronic pain patients tend to be overly solicitous, to beseech, to implore or feign gratitude when they feel indignation. They do this because they are afraid they will not get the treatment they need.

Often, that treatment is an opioid analgesic. Abuse, prejudice, and ignorance have put a strong stigma on this class of medication, adding to the pain patient's woes. While most patients on a regimen of opioid analgesics report overwhelming relief, some still regard these medications with suspicion, failing to understand the important distinction between tolerance, physical dependence, and addiction. Tolerance is the body's need for an increasing quantity of a medication in order to achieve the same therapeutic effect. Physical dependence, by contrast, is a known effect of certain types of medication and is characterized by symptoms of withdrawal that differ among medicines, be they sleep aids, opioid analgesics, blood pressure medications (some of which result in physical dependence and some of which do not), or the caffeine in our daily cup of joe. Medically speaking, physical dependence it is not considered to be either positive or negative.

Addiction is a different issue entirely. It is a primary, chronic, disease influenced by psychosocial and environmental factors. It is also strongly genetic. Addicts are not made from people who do not have the appropriate genetic makeup. Exposure to pain medications, or to alcohol, for that matter, does not create addicts. Addiction requires more than that. It is a biological affliction that demands, at least, both exposure and predisposition. Pseudoaddiction is a syndrome in which patients who desperately seek relief from an undertreated pain mimic the behavior of those seeking drugs for different reasons, and this merely clouds the picture. *People in genuine chronic pain suffer the more because these distinctions are not generally understood.*

Whatever the organic cause of the pain or the mode of treatment, the voices that follow ring with courage and demand compassion. They are the voices of the young and the old, from accidents and disease, from all walks of life, but most of all they are the voices of people in pain.

Mary Vargas, J.D.

❧

Mary Vargas, a Washington, D.C.–area attorney, works as an advocate for deaf people who have been wronged by the health care and legal systems. She is twenty-eight years old, and a chronic pain patient.

I understand your pain is the result of a car accident.

I was in law school in Connecticut when it happened. I had a friend visiting and there was nothing but *Baywatch* on television, so we took a drive to White's Flower Farm. I was waiting to turn into the farm and the lady who was driving behind me hit me. She said she never even saw me. She said she was looking at the scenery. My car was pushed off the road and ended up facing the opposite direction—a stone wall on one side of it, a telephone pole on the other. We were very, very lucky.

So this was a whiplash injury?

Yes. When it happened, I thought it was no big deal. I wanted it to go away, thought it would go away. The doctor said sometimes these things last six months. Six months came to an end, I was planning a backpacking trip to Germany—we were planning all kinds of normal life activities—and life was getting *less* normal by the minute rather than *more* normal by the minute.

So the pain was getting worse?

Much worse.

4

So it wasn't bad right away?

I knew immediately there was a problem. The car stopped, and I remember realizing that there was music playing. I didn't know we had crashed. My friend said we had been hit and told me the car was still moving, and I put on the brakes. I felt this burning on the side of my face. I went to the emergency room a few hours later. The pain was much worse by the time I got there.

You didn't go right away in an ambulance?

No. No I didn't. I didn't think I needed to. I was able to stand up, I was able to move, I wasn't bleeding anywhere. I went home, got a rental car, drove the rental car to the hospital. So they told me there was some straightening of my spine, whiplash. You know, whiplash is portrayed in a suspicious light in the United States. I don't think it necessarily helped that I was a law student talking about a whiplash injury. That was the beginning of visits to thirteen or fourteen different doctors over a period of years, trying to figure out what was going on.

And what was the eventual diagnosis?

Ultimately it was suboccipital neuralgia. But the diagnosis was never really very important.

Not very important because there was no specific treatment for it, or because it sounds like another way of saying you have pain in your neck? Frankly, it sounds more like a description than a diagnosis.

Well, that's exactly it. The pain is what is most important. At that point, I had been to so many different doctors, had so many different procedures that I was glad to have a term that meant they believed me.

Are you implying that other, earlier doctors didn't believe you?

Nobody ever said that they didn't believe me. But I had a sense that they wondered, "What's the big deal? Is it really that bad? Maybe you just have a really low threshold of pain."

Do you have a low pain threshold?

I don't know. I don't think so. I don't know what to compare it to.

Nor do I. I'm not sure what the phrase means. My wife tells me that if I gave birth, I would die. Maybe that means she thinks my pain threshold is low. Did they do tests to explore your experience?

They did X rays, they did MRIs, and then we got into this murky area of tests that they said also might *help*. Tests that themselves might actually help me feel better, nerve blocks and the like. I went through a lot of that.

Were the tests conclusive in any way?

My husband and I were always the 1 percent. They always said there was a very small percentage of side effects, but everything right along the way seemed to happen to us. I had a procedure called prolotherapy done in New York City. It is something used with athletes. Irritants are injected into your muscles to cause them to break down and build up scar tissue to strengthen the injured area. The idea was that these irritants would be injected into my neck and it would become stronger and the pain would be less. The first time I went in for that therapy, they hit a nerve. I was paralyzed on one side of my body. This isn't the kind of injury you can see easily on a test. It seems like a lot of times the tests don't show things. They certainly didn't for me.

Were you injury prone as a young girl? Did you fall off a horse, walk into a door, that sort of thing?

I never walked into a door. I was never sick when I was a kid. I danced. Ballet was an important part of my life. I ended up stopping because of problems with my feet, but other than that there was nothing.

How did your friends and family respond to you having pain as the re-sult of a car accident?

I was throwing up. I was ill from the pain. It was obvious that I was hurting, but there was no visible manifestation of my injury. My husband didn't know how bad it was. At the beginning, it was very much just me going to the doctor, me going to the phys-ical therapist. At some point he realized that this problem wasn't going away. It was having a huge impact on our lives. It became more both of us going to appointments. In some ways, it was more him doing the research on what treatments were out there and what doctors provided pain care, those kinds of things.

Did the pain become a third partner in your marriage?

That's exactly what my husband said.

It had a personality of its own, a presence of its own?

It was more that the pain negated my own personality than that it brought a new personality to the marriage. The pain took over to the extent that anything that was extra in my life we didn't do. I went to work, I went home, I went to bed—if I wasn't throwing up on the bathroom floor. We didn't go to the mall, we didn't camp, we didn't go on trips.

Not much fun.

No.

How did your marriage change?

We married a week before I started law school. We hadn't even been married a year when I had the accident.

So you were still in the process of defining what the marriage was.

Very much so. It made it stronger.

How do people outside your immediate family respond to your pain?

They tend not to know about it. I don't really feel comfortable telling them about it. I think my boss would be shocked to know that during litigation, when we were in court, I went to the bathroom and got sick. (*crying*) He would be shocked. But you said outside of my immediate family. My immediate family is my husband. My parents' reaction to it was really shocking to me. Not so much their reaction to the whole medical process and how I was feeling, but their reaction to me starting to talk about was very negative. They said things like "Do you really want people to know that?"

And yet they know of your propensity for advocacy. They know about the role of moral outrage in your life. They must have known this about you for some time. So it must be a privacy issue. Is that it?

It's more like talking about pain is somehow embarrassing. My family came over on the *Mayflower*. They were the second ones to step off. The Winslows. Theirs was the first marriage in the New World. Talk about Puritans.

Amazing! So do you think talking about pain is embarrassing for most people?

Yes.

And why do you think that is?

People have a sense that they are supposed to have a stiff upper lip. To just deal with it. Mind over matter. You can convince yourself it isn't that bad. If you looked like you were Stoic, standing mutely and working, invincible, that you could make it come true, that you could make yourself better.

What do you do for the pain?

I have been on a lot of different medications. Currently, I use an opioid patch and a spinal cord stimulator, which has a huge role. The stimulator has electrodes implanted in my neck where the pain is, and wires run down my lower back where there is a battery implanted under my skin. The battery sends electrical impulses to the electrodes at the back of my head to cover the pain impulses, which for some reason are being sent to my brain. A computer chip controls it, and I can make minor changes with a device that looks like a remote control. The battery has to be replaced from time to time.

You are quite young, but when you were even younger, when you were a little girl wondering how life would be, did you ever imagine that pain would play such a role?

No. Why would I? You don't even know what pain is until it happens to you. I mean, you can watch it, you can see somebody suffering and register that experience in your own way, but until it is actually you and yours, you can't understand it. One of the things that I deal with a lot in my real life—my job—is the question of what it means to be a person with a disability. There is a question whether someone who suffers pain is a person with a disability. I think the answer is easy. Of course they are.

You just referred to your job as your "real life." Most people would not call their job their real life.

I meant my grown-up life.

Let's stay with "real life" for just a Freudian moment. Is it possible that the experience of being not busy, intellectually, makes you more vulnerable to your discomfort, so you do what so many of us do, which is to keep busy sometimes, to not feel a variety of pains? Did this car accident you had, and the pain that ensued, change the balance between your work and your private life?

Being busy doesn't make the pain go away, but as far as shifting the balance of things, I would say that I'm pretty much a Type A personality, someone who expects a lot of herself, and having this pain is pretty humbling. There are some things that I can't do that I used to be able to do, and some things that we can't change.

After that first prolotherapy that paralyzed my left side, I told them for hours that I couldn't feel my arm or my leg. They told me that they didn't know why, but that the problem would go away. Later that day, there was some speculation that they might have hit my spinal cord during the procedure.

Suddenly there was malpractice on the horizon.

There sure was. And they wanted to start me on antibiotics just in case. One of the hardest things about pain is that when you are hurting you can't be an advocate for yourself. My husband, who is an attorney, too, became my advocate. One of the doctors started to hook up the IV for an antibiotic, even though we had said we wanted to find out for sure what was going on first, and my husband jumped up and grabbed the medication and said, "No! Not until you know what is going on!"

So your husband helps you cope with your pain?

My husband is very much the voice of reason. He doesn't live my pain, but he knows how it affects my life and his own. He always says that his role is to bear witness—having someone bear witness somehow gives meaning to suffering where there is no meaning otherwise. After we had been to many doctors together, he took over the role of detailing and explaining my accident, my injury and my problems, because I was just too occupied with fighting my pain to go over and over it. By the way, do you read Stephen King?

Not much.

Well, earlier you asked me about pain having a presence. Stephen King wrote a book called *Dreamcatcher*, and in that book he describes these beings that take over a person's body. The personality remains inside the person's body as if locked in a small room, while the "intruder" takes over interactions with the world. That is exactly what pain is like. You are relegated to a back corner of your mind while some survival instinct takes over to keep you functioning day to day. Incidentally, one of the characters in *Dreamcatcher* is recovering from having been hit by a car. King himself was hit by a car and badly hurt, and, I could tell when I saw him on TV, angry about the whole thing, which surprised some people but I found it appropriate. It's as if he put his pain on paper in his book.

I can tell that you are angry, too. Did you sue the woman who hit you?
Yes.

Did the settlement help your anger?
A little, but it wasn't a direct connection. What helped was the settlement conference before a judge. The other side said my pain couldn't have been bad because I did things like decorate a Christmas tree, graduate at the top of my law school class, get a fellowship and hold down a job. Imagine trying to use against me the fact that I pressed through the pain to do things that were important to me. The judge saw things my way, and it was a vindication, a kind of justice more powerful than the financial settlement. It validated the fact that I had survived, chosen a hard path and kept going.

If I were to ask you to rank validation and relief from physical pain, which would come first?
It would depend upon on how bad the pain is at the time you asked me.

That suggests that validation is awfully important, that it answers the emotional aspects of chronic pain the way palliative procedures, medication and devices answer the physical side.
Once you are in pain, your ability to cope with things, even

things that should be simple, is lessened. The validation that you are talking about helps, but it doesn't solve the underlying problem that got you there to begin with—the pain.

Compassion, then?
Compassion is an easier word to agree to than validation.

What do you get out of compassion?
It goes back to acknowledging that there is something that is wrong that you can't change, having someone bear witness. You don't have to work through it alone. For example, when I come home from work and feel too sick to do anything but climb into bed, it is important that my husband sees that I feel awful, that he recognizes the pain without my having to explain it.

I remember going to many doctors who told me to learn to live with the pain. One doctor told me it was like diabetes or heart disease, and that lots of people learn to live with those diseases. My husband I always maintained that pain was different—and it is. I don't feel that I have accepted pain as inevitable—don't get me wrong, it isn't something you can change by just wishing it away—but rather something that modern medicine can address if patients and families fight for a solution.

Hertz Nazaire

ের

Hertz Nazaire is an artist. He is twenty-eight years old, and suffers from sickle-cell anemia. I interview him in his apartment building in Bridgeport, Connecticut.

Do you think of yourself as a person in pain?
I think of myself as an artist. That's how I define myself. That's the thing that keeps me going.

What medium do you work in?
Mostly oil pastels. Some acrylics. Bright colors.

What is the source of your chronic pain?
Sickle-cell anemia. I was born with it. I've had it all my life.

What is your first memory of pain?
I remember my mother rocking me back and forth to make me feel better when I was a baby. The subtle movement was like a meditation. It had a calming effect on me. I was born in Haiti. There was no medication available there, not even an aspirin, so I just had to deal with the pain I went through as a child. It was awful then and it is awful now. The difference is, now I manage my pain, but in Haiti things were really different.

Is the pain throughout your body, or is it mostly in a particular place?
Sometimes in the joints, sometimes in the chest—anywhere that I have a blood vessel. If it happens in the brain, I get a stroke.

What causes the pain?

A normal red blood cell is supposed to be round. Sickle-cell anemia changes it into a half-moon shape. My blood cells are no longer round and soft. They're sickle-shaped and hard, and they get stuck in veins. When they get stuck, the area gets blocked, the oxygen doesn't get to the tissue, the tissue starts to suffocate, and that causes pain. That's how it happens.

How were you treated by friends and family when you complained of pain as a little boy?

I was treated as different. My mother was very overprotective. I wasn't supposed to join the Boy Scouts, although I *did* join them, but I wasn't allowed to go on the field trips, which are really a big part of the scouts. I didn't play any sports. Mostly I hit the books and did my art. I've been painting since I was a little kid. It's been my best friend.

What images do you paint?

All kinds of things, but in everything I use vibrant, bright colors. With depression you feel dark gray colors, and I like to put any kind of image that comes to mind on black paper, but in very bright colors, very vibrant colors that I remember from outdoor tropical places like Haiti.

Animals?

Not really, although there was a lady that wanted a teddy bear drawn.

Did you have a teddy bear as a little boy?

I had a few. I still get them even now. When I spend time in the hospital, teddy bears are some of the comforting things that people bring with them when they come to see me. I still have them all over my place, all over my room.

How often do you go to the hospital?

It varies. Sometimes it's no more than twice a year, but there was a three-year period when I was in the hospital for ten months out of the year. Sometime I get sick but I take care of myself at home. Everyone at the hospital knows me, because I've been going to the same hospital since I was a child.

How old were you when you came to the United States?

I was nine.

Did you come with your folks?

My mother was here before I was. She was an immigrant in New York, and it would have been difficult to bring me along at the beginning because I was sick. The doctors always told her that I would die before I got to the age of eighteen. She left me in Haiti and came here searching for a dream, and when the dream happened, she sent for me. She died in a car accident when she was in her thirties and I was fourteen. I was in the car. She was my safety, my comfort. That loss is an important part of my life. It's something that I have to live with.

Tell me about the accident.

We were going food shopping. We were on the Merrit Parkway here in Connecticut. It was August 31. The car lost control and we hit a tree on the side and that was it. My sister was in the back seat with me. She flew to the windshield and came back and landed in my lap. I was awake through everything. These images kind of stay with you.

How is your sister?

She was in a coma for a while, but now she's all right. We have different fathers, so after that happened her father kept her but decided he couldn't raise a son with sickle-cell—have someone so sick around. So I went to the state, and then I went to live with a godmother of mine.

What about your own father?
I met him once in 1986, in Haiti. He was an English teacher there, a prominent man. I'm not even sure if he's alive now. The last time I talked to him was back when my mom died.

So your godmother raised you?
I was already fourteen, so just through high school. Then I went off to college.

Where did you go to high school?
At West Hills, in Stamford, Connecticut.

And college?
I wanted to follow the arts thing. I made the mistake of going to the Art Institute of Fort Lauderdale. I wanted to get away from the winters, and I liked the colors down there in Florida. I love colors. I use those colors in my heart.

Why was it a mistake?
I wanted to try and get into graphic design or illustration, something that would allow me to use my art in a professional way and make a living. That was the goal. That was the plan. Florida turned out to be a mistake because pain management in Florida seemed like the worst in the country. It was terrible. I was getting sick left and right because they didn't manage my pain. So it was a mistake to go there on the basis of my health. I didn't realize that I needed to pay so much attention to my pain, to manage it that carefully.

I just wanted to be a normal kid. I just wanted to follow my dreams. But having a chronic illness, you really need your doctor to back you up. I didn't realize how much I needed my doctor's help. For the first two years down there I was in the honors group. I got straight As. I was doing great, but working at the same time and going to school made me sick. I was holding down three jobs just to pay for school. I still have to pay off $42,000 in loans. I dropped out after the second year because I just couldn't handle it any more. I got sick too much. I was in the intensive care unit many times with acute-chest syndrome—pain that could kill me.

What is acute–chest syndrome?

Sickle-cell damages organs because you're sick all the time. When you get pneumonia a lot and the lungs collapse and there are complications, that's acute chest syndrome. That happened to me many times, but I survived it. Twice, I survived my heart stopping. There are so many things that happen with sickle-cell that I can't think about next week because although I'm sitting here today, I'm not sure when I'll next get sick. I could get sick tonight. I could get sick two hours from now, or I could get sick next week. It's very hard to plan what you have going on.

There are many people with sickle-cell that live a relatively normal life, getting sick say once every year or two. They can manage. They can become nurses, doctors, lawyers, whatever they want. But there are some of us who have pain more chronically. It stays with us, and our quality of life is a bit different. The pain is very strong, and you can't do anything when you're in crisis. Women who have sickle-cell claim that the pain is ten times worse than childbirth pain. That's what they say in support groups. That's what I've heard many times from friends of mine. It's a very strong pain. You can't really function when you're suffering like that.

Tell me about the support groups.

I've headed a few support groups, but it is difficult to get people to come and talk. A lot of people just don't want to talk about things that are so private and deeply rooted. Maybe their pride won't let them. Maybe they don't want to complain. For me, a black person from Haiti, I find that your parents instill a certain strength in you when you're growing up. You're taught that you have to fight to get what you want, fight to get where you're going. You have to fight the society you live in. You have to fight prejudices. You have to fight for everything. You can't sit down and complain about things you can't control, so maybe you don't seek help as much as you should. You try to do things on your own all the time.

It sounds as if your mom gave you a lot.

She did. A lot of my strength comes from her. It's not that she really *told* me how to behave, but more how my suffering affected her. She worked two jobs to pay the bills and had to get up at four A.M. to carry me down to the car and off to the hospital and then stay there until six or seven o'clock and then go off to work. Sometimes I stopped complaining because I didn't want to see her hurt.

You try not to put your pain out there because you want to protect others, especially the ones you care about. I really dislike people feeling sorry for me. I want to be normal. I want to have a normal life. I want to follow my dreams and everything. I tell these stories because I want others to understand how to manage their pain and manage their care. In the telling, I'm putting myself out in public and that doesn't feel all that great to me when I come back home and when I have to sleep, because it reminds me every day that I'm living with this.

Tell me about your dreams.

Basically getting off disability, getting off food stamps or other things the government supplies. Avoiding being homeless, and some of the other things that have happened to me. I want the American dream that my mother came here for and worked and sacrificed to get. Everything I do, I do because I want to realize the dreams that she had. I want to live as I can despite what I have to go through. I've been working on my art. That's positive. I could have let so many negative things into my life.

Is this building where we are talking housing for the disabled?
This is a supported-living facility. They have a support structure for people who have different types of issues. But it's an apartment building.

Do you consider the other folks who live here your community, your extended family?
I'm not that public a person. Actually, I'm very private. I'm never in the public areas of this building. I stick to myself most of the time. I talk to a few people, and that's it. People see me as an artist, walking in or out with a painting, or they see me on TV talking about sickle-cell for the local sickle-cell organization. Or they see me in the newspaper. But I'm very private because I need it. I'm not very comfortable being out. When I lost my mother, that was it. You asked about support structure. I haven't had a family since I was fourteen, so I really don't understand that structure.

You were with your godmother.
That experience was all about learning to cope with abuse. She was very abusive verbally. Letting people inside, trusting them, that's hard for me. I had trouble trusting doctors for a while. For a long while, I didn't trust them at all.

Did you think they had some agenda other than to help you?
In pediatrics, when I was a little child, everything was great. The nurses cared; there was a toy room; there were all these doctors

hovering over me all the time. People don't want to see a child in pain. But as soon as I turned eighteen, became an adolescent, moved on to a regular hospital floor, things changed. People treated me differently.

They regarded your pain differently?

They regarded me as a *person* differently. It felt as soon as I stepped into the emergency room that judgment was passed against me. There's a stigma attached to sickle-cell patients. It's like they thought I was seeking drugs. They didn't believe I was in pain. There's so much stuff on the street but they still seemed to think I was coming to the hospital for a vacation or to get high. I'm not sure if it's a race thing or what.

One time the ambulance picked me up. I was only wearing a T-shirt and shorts—what I had been wearing to bed. They sedated me. When I woke up, still in extreme pain, they told me it was time to go home. They didn't believe I was in enough pain to be admitted, didn't believe I had any real problems. I couldn't walk. I was sitting in a chair in the emergency room and a security guard came out and said, "You have to leave." He was very serious about it. It was snowing and I had no one to call, but they put me out on the street. That was here in Bridgeport.

Do you have friends now on whom you can rely?

I have relationships with the local sickle-cell organization. I volunteer through them, do health fairs, try and help other people that have sickle-cell like me. That group is my support structure. The director over there is like a mother to me. She goes beyond the call of duty when it comes to caring for people with sickle-cell. We have a tight relationship.

The most important thing for me is to get a positive message out to people out there, kids growing up with this feeling of hopelessness, people who are not being treated well by their family and are afraid of what is happening to them, afraid they might die. Sometimes I have to worry about where my money's going to come from, what I'm going to eat the next day, how I'm going to pay my bills, whether I'm going to be out on the street the next day. Still, I manage to hope and pray and keep a positive outlook. Hope is important to me. I look for hope in everything that I do. I'm still hoping for a cure, that some day I won't have to deal with this. People have to know that they can survive this. More than survive. They can get it all, everything that they want and desire. It's very important that they know that.

Allyson Gabrey

∞

Allyson Gabrey is a pain patient. I interview her at her home in Port St. Lucie, Florida. She makes me some coffee. Her kids busy themselves in the other room. Occasionally they come to check on their mother.

I understand that there has been quite a bit of suffering in your family.
Well, my mother is a diabetic. She had her leg amputated. It took fifty staples. They took it off above the knee because the circulation had frozen up. She'd been in the ICU [Intensive Care Unit] for three days. They moved her to the a regular room, but still hadn't given her pain medication. They arranged for her breakfast, but not for any pain medication. So I stopped the doctor in the hallway and asked, "Are you going to give my mother any pain medication?" He answered, "Well, the leg's been cut off. It can't hurt anymore." I literally grabbed him by the arm and said, "She has fifty staples in her leg. When was the last time you had *your* leg cut off? How do *you* know how she feels? You're going to give my mother pain medication, and you're going to give it to her now." I really felt like I was ready to wrestle this doctor to the ground if he didn't give my mother pain medication. My mother's a tough woman. For her to lie there and cry, she had to be in pain. He was worried about her becoming addicted, but he wrote the order out. Believe me, addiction was the least of my mother's concerns at the time.

How much longer did your mother live after that?
Four years.

Now you yourself are on pain medication. Why is that?
I have spinal stenosis, and two herniated discs in my neck, and three in my lumber spine that press on the S–1 nerve root and shoot pain down to my leg. It's very intense pain. Living in Florida, I don't know what it is, but when storms move in, as they do every day in summer, it makes the pain increase. I can't tell you why, but I know when a storm's coming. Barometric pressure, I guess.

Have you had surgery on your back?
Surgery is out of the question.

Really?
The doctor said that scar tissue damage could cause just as much damage if not more. My condition will lead to paralysis eventually. Should it progress faster than normal, then the doctor would consider surgery, but it's such a delicate area around the spinal cord that he doesn't want to mess with it.

Were you able to get adequate pain relief pretty much right away when you went to the doctor?
I went through a period of time when they gave me weaker-end pain medication. They acted like it should be enough, but it wasn't. I finally went to an internal medicine doctor. They wanted me to go see a neurologist, but I'm uninsurable, and I couldn't afford his fees. Turns out it doesn't matter anyway, because nothing can be done for me except pain management. That's what they told me—that physical therapy was out, that surgery was out, pain management was all they could offer.

The first time the doctor offered me an opioid I said no. Then the pain got so bad, when she offered it to me again I said I'd try it. I couldn't believe the relief. It was like I didn't have the spinal stenosis. The doctor warned me to remember my back injury, not to think I was superwoman and go back to doing the work I was doing before. I used to do landscaping with my husband. I mowed lawns, I cut trees, I trimmed bushes, I did all that stuff. She warned me not to try it anymore.

How old are your children?
Nineteen, ten, and four.

Before you had your pain adequately controlled, was your interaction affected?
My interaction with my children was nothing. I lay on the couch with my heating pad, and the kids just tore through the house, destroying it. I would sit on the chair and get up to cook, sit back down, then do the dishes. The littlest one would sit with me, and I would watch cartoons with her so I could keep an eye on her. I kept her toys out here so I could keep an eye on her. My back was too painful for me to do anything else.

Is your husband managing the business without you?
He had to hire another guy, so it put him back some.

Your brother has a back problem as well, is that right?
My brother had two rods put in his back. A month after the surgery, he was in a car accident that bent those rods in his back. He'd gone back to work a month early and he was driving and this lady pulled out in front of him. He was a painter. He was on his way back from work. A fifty-pound sprayer and all his equipment came forward in the van and hit him hard enough to actually bend those metal rods. So after a long period of time on weaker medications he started on opioids. Now, with any narcotic, over a period of time your body does become dependent on it. That comes with it. Nothing you can do about that.

They weren't giving him enough. He was still in pain. Finally he went to a pain center, and they put a morphine pump in him. Well, that morphine pump failed while my mother was living with my brother, and dying. The pump was blowing up and blowing up. We told him to go to the hospital, but he said, "I'm not leaving Ma. I'm not leaving my mother." Finally, the pump literally exploded. Burst right out of him, fell on the floor. They told him he was lucky it did—that the infection would have killed him in a few days if it hadn't been able to drain. They put him on a long-acting opioid pill and then more pills for break-through pain. My brother was literally a cripple. He walked with two canes. This was the same man who played softball every day after work. Rollerbladed. Played hockey. It's bad enough he had this life-changing accident, but to have to continue to suffer was just terrible.

So he went into the pharmacy with the prescription after the pump burst, and the pharmacist gave him back his prescription and told him, "You have a problem in your house, and I'm not filling this." So my brother lifted up his shirt and showed him where he was bleeding and started at yelling at them, "I just had a pump explode and I just lost my mother and now I've got you giving me crap about a pill?"

Are the pharmacists the only folks you've found who have that kind of prejudice?

I've found doctors who are afraid to write the medication. Before I found my doctor, I would go to the hospital and they would give me a prescription for five or so low-strength tablets. I mean, that's not going to do me much good.

They knew that your pain would continue after the five tablets were gone, but they wouldn't give you any more?

They were worried that I was going to be dependent, and I understand that. I am dependent. I smoke cigarettes, too, and I'm dependent on the nicotine. But I'm more dependent upon being pain free.

You use the word "dependent" instead of the word "addicted."
You're right. There's a difference, and it's clear to me. I'm addicted to nicotine, but I'm dependent on my pain medications. Without my medications, my pain would be intolerable. I wouldn't be able to care for my children, wouldn't be able to care for my home. I don't want to spend the rest of my life lying on the couch. Why should I?

Do you experience any prejudice now?
Since I started on the opioids, I even experience it from my husband. I mean, he didn't like seeing me in pain, he didn't like having to pick up the slack, didn't like seeing the house a mess. He notices a difference now, but he's worried about the pills. He keeps saying, "I want you off these, I want you off these." And I say, "So you want me back to where you're gonna have to come home early and take care of the kids? You want me to suffer because of the bad press that's been given to certain drugs."

What's his response?
He doesn't have a response. My whole neighborhood knows I'm on an opioid. They do treat me differently because of it. They've heard stories on the news. When I go into a pharmacy, if I'm looking for an antibiotic and they don't have it, they will call around and find it for me. If I bring in a prescription for an opioid, they fling it back at me and tell me they don't have it. I ask where I'm going to get it, then, and they tell me they don't know. So I say, "Excuse me, but this is the time that I'm supposed to have this filled. I'm not in here two weeks early trying to scam you—I'm following the doctor's directions, I'm sticking with one

pharmacy." I get this attitude from the pharmacies. Last month I actually had to *leave town* to get my prescription filled. Went to Palm City. That's in another county. I got no attitude there. None at all.

It seems like we're dealing with two kinds of prejudice: one against people who take these medications, and another against people who are in pain.

If you complain, you're a crybaby. My husband said that to me one time. I had to remind him that I had all three children with no pain relievers at all. I walked around working with a collapsed lung for a week before I went to the hospital. People told me it was anxiety, 'cause it was inventory time. Ha! A crybaby I am not! I've always had a very strong tolerance to pain. The doctor I have now, she's great. She gives me my medicine. Her philosophy is: Why be in pain when you don't have to be? That's the philosophy all doctors should have, but they don't. If you have records showing you have problems, you should be given what you need. That's a doctor's job, isn't it? To heal? To relieve suffering? That's their oath, isn't it? But they're more worried about what the DEA is going to think, or what their reputation in town is going to be. They're worried that they're going to be known as a drug doctor. Truly, I don't know what their problem is.

Hal E. Garner Jr.

☙

Hal Garner was a promising young star with the Buffalo Bills football team when a field injury ended his career. He then began an odyssey in search of pain relief that cost him his home, his property, custody of his children, his marriage, and left him a pariah in his community. I meet with him at his home in Logan, Utah.

Tell me a bit about yourself.

I was born in Baton Rouge, Louisiana, and grew up here in Logan, Utah. My dad was a football player at Utah State and I wanted to be like him. From fourth grade on, I told myself I was going to be a professional football player. I did what it took, every day, to fulfill my dream. I read, I studied, I practiced, I worked out. I wanted to become a hero to myself, to my father, and to other professional athletes.

When I was eleven years old, I ran through a plate glass window at a friend's house. I suffered lacerations and I tore tendons in my feet. They told me I would never be able to run again, that I would drag a foot. I wouldn't accept that fact. I was in a wheelchair for six months, and I did physical therapy. By the end of that summer, I was playing league football. I was in tears afterward from the pain, but I did what nobody believed I could do.

In junior high I had a knee injury, and in high school I had several more, including several concussions and broken bones—things I could live with. I got a scholarship from Logan High

28

School to Utah State University, where I had a great career, although I went through two more knee surgeries playing. They told me again that I would end my career there, but the more people tell me I can't do something the more I want to prove them wrong, even if I have to force myself past my limits and hurt myself. My dad came into the hospital and told me I'd never play professional ball, and I told him "Bullshit."

I was 6 feet 4 inches, 225 pounds, and I had the triangle numbers—height, weight and speed. I was faster than most everybody, I consistently ran 4.4s in the forty-yard dash. I was All-Conference, All-American, and then I got drafted to the Buffalo Bills, sixth pick in the third round. I didn't want to go, because Minnesota and Buffalo were the two worst teams in the two coldest places, but a buddy of mine got drafted, too, and I figured it was okay so I went.

Things went pretty well. My second year, I won the starting job. Fourth game into the season, I blew out my knee again. I had knee and ankle surgery, and thumb and turf-toe operations. The team wasn't doing that well, and I retired after four years in the NFL. I came home and went into construction because that was what my dad did, and I operated heavy equipment. I wasn't happy. I was still young, and I wanted to play football. I called the Bills head coach and asked him for a chance to come back. He said, "Hal, you know people can't retire and then come back to the NFL. It doesn't happen." I asked him for the opportunity to prove him wrong. I went through a lot of physical therapy to get my knees strong and I proved him wrong and made the team. I played for two more years and then we went to the Super Bowl. It was a good choice on my part. After five weeks of training camp, preparing for my seventh year with the Bills, in the last segment of the last day of the last week of training, my friend Jim

Kelly, the quarterback, placed himself in the huddle where I could read his lips. It was a goal-line situation. It was a quick, one-step, drop back pass. When the ball was snapped I stepped back and jumped as high as I could and blocked the pass. The offensive tackle grabbed my shoulders and slammed me down to try and save the pass and my knee didn't bend, and my back buckled.

I felt a pop, pop, pop. The doctors fed me full of an anti-inflammatory and painkillers and told me that if I didn't play in the last game in the preseason, I wouldn't make the team. From my perspective, they just wanted to get me on film so it would be hard for me to sue them for disability. They gave me painkillers before the game, but my coach could see I was dragging my leg and was in pain, and he didn't like that and he pulled me. He got reprimanded for it. The next day the head coach called me down and they fired me.

I got in contact with a well-known Buffalo attorney and went in for an MRI and X rays. The doctor told me there was nothing wrong and told me to sign a paper saying so. I wouldn't. I flew home and went to the University of Utah Health Services Center and had them do an MRI, which showed two severely herniated discs. I fought the Bills in court for two years—a battle of attrition, the big guy against the little guy—to win disability, and salary for the year in which I was injured. I ran up big legal bills—I had tests with specialists in San Diego, Florida, Rutgers, San Francisco. They said I had a strong case. I went back to Buffalo and I won.

I gather that wasn't the end of your troubles.

No. After the court case, I had my back operated on. Two years later I was picking up my two-year-old son and I felt a pop in my back and I was back in bed and I had another surgery. A year later my wife and I were picking up a piece of heavy glass and I felt another pop. That led to another surgery. From 1991 to 1998 I was in level-six to level-nine [on a scale of one to ten] pain, but nobody would help me. Even the doctors at the University of Utah would only give me so much medication and would only refill it so many times.

Level-ten pain is unbearable?
You want to kill yourself. Bone pain can only go to level four. Spinal cord pain can go all the way. Level ten can even cause paralysis.

Looking at all your history since childhood, I have to wonder why you would keep exposing yourself to injury.
For the excitement, I suppose. The thrill. The money. The glory. The limelight. I love professional sports.

Was it worth it?
Hell no, it wasn't worth it.

Would you do it again?
(*smiling ruefully*) In a heartbeat.

Tell me about your attempts to live a normal life.
Nobody wanted to help me with my pain. That was the big thing. They didn't want to give me drugs. They said they couldn't. I ran into prejudices at every job I went to, I was seen as addicted to medications. This is a small town, and everybody thought they knew what was going on with me, but nobody really understood what I was going through, trying to live in a conservative valley, being married and having two children, running four businesses. I owned two pawnshops, a grocery store, and was a bail bondsman—a bounty hunter. It was intolerable to be perceived as an addict—to have people look at me the way they

did. I was the star growing up, and suddenly I was seen as a drug-ridden freak.

I had to paint a smile on my face every day and pretend that I was not in pain. I went from being a professional athlete who could do anything to not being able jump an inch off the ground and play basketball with my son. Everyone gets sick of hearing about how much you hurt, see? Nobody understands it, so they don't want to listen to it. They think you're making it up. They want you to see a psychiatrist. But this pain is real. It comes from rods in my back, from scar tissue from surgeries suffocating and pressing on nerves. It was so hard to sleep, to get out of bed in the morning, to work day to day and make a living and keep everybody happy.

The medications they were using fogged me up, and the dosages had side effects that made me look like a heroin addict. I said, "I can't keep this up. I'm going to die." I stopped eating for two weeks. I stopped going to the bathroom for two weeks. Their way of treating me was slowly killing me. Finally, I woke up in the morning from a dream in which my mother, who died of cancer, was telling me to do something about the way things were going. So I did. I put myself in the hospital. That's what I had to do in order to get the pump, which puts medication directly into the spinal cord. No side effects, no toxicity or shakes and sweats and shivers, just pain relief. I learned that from the specialists at the NFL Players Association.

So, finally, after eight years your pain is satisfactorily managed?
My life is 50 to 75 percent better. A pain specialist came to town and opened a clinic, and saved my life. Now I don't have to paint a smile on my face, and I don't have to make excuses for myself. I'm not addicted to anything, I'm simply dependent on my medication for pain relief. I need it, but I'm not obsessed by it. Without it, I'd die. Without it, I'd kill myself.

But all that was too late to save your marriage?

When I was in the hospital that last time, my wife couldn't handle it anymore. She couldn't stay up one more night watching me, afraid I was going to die. She left, and she took my kids, my horses, the dream ranch I bought while I was in the NFL. The worst thing was losing my kids. It was almost as bad as all the physical pain I've been through. I won joint physical custody, which means I get to keep them half the time, but when I went to a psychologist friend of mine and asked him what was best for the kids he said it was better for them to have more stability and a place they could call home. So now I get to see them every other weekend and one night a week, even though they live only half a mile away. I want to be involved with them, to see them, to hold them, to pick them up from school, but that's not what's best for them, not on an equal-time basis. I feel like I live in a bubble and my kids are outside it and I can't talk to them. (*crying*) I can't hold them and I can't hug them.

If I were to ask your wife, what would she say about you?

That I was mentally abusive. That I was physically abusive. That I was suicidal—a drug addict. No good.

All because of the pain?

All because of the heavy burden of it. And the fact that I couldn't get the relief.

Until it was too late.

That's right.

Is it better with the kids now?

Sure. They love me. They don't believe all the things people say about me. They know what I'm like. They know I just want to be happy. They call me every night to tell me they love me. We love each other more every day.

Esther Reiter

❧

Seventeen years ago, pain patient Esther Reiter suffered a stroke caused by an arteriovenous malformation of the thalamus of her brain. A Chicago resident, she visits Memorial-Sloan Kettering in New York City for treatment of the resultant thalamic pain. I interview her in a small and featureless treatment room at that hospital.

Tell me about thalamic pain.

It affects the left side of my body, the left hand and arm, followed by the face and then the leg. I feel it most in the left arm and hand. When the pain first started, I was unaware of what was happening. I didn't know it was a result of the stroke. I had never heard of thalamic pain. I thought that when you had a stroke you were paralyzed, and then you worked hard in rehab, and then it was over. I did all those things, and then three months later I was struck by this terrible pain. Initially, the pain was bearable.

Among the medications most often used seventeen years ago were antidepressants. The side effects at that time—grogginess, dry mouth, constipation in the extreme—were worse than the pain itself. Antidepressants used today aren't as extreme in their side effects, but the one I was put on then was, and I had difficulty dealing with it. I thought it would be better for me to manage the pain than the side effects. Over the next two years, the pain increased to a point at which I wasn't managing it well. I was

34

functional—I went to work every day—but I was in a lot of pain and doing a lot of suffering. It was then that I was given the diagnosis—thalamic pain.

Thalamic pain comes in different sizes and shapes, and it's not the same every day. One of the pains is a feeling of tightening of muscles. In me it feels like I'm trying to make a fist. The muscles don't necessarily actually tighten, but the message that the brain sends is that the muscle is tight. So I went to try biofeedback. It allowed me to relax my muscles, but the problem was it was only effective when I concentrated on it. The minute I went on with my daily life, the biofeedback was no longer effective. I asked the therapist "When will the time come when I can do two things at once?" He answered that it would take about twenty years of practice. That's the most difficult part of biofeedback or meditation. While you're doing it it's effective, but there are no lasting long term effects of these practices in terms of controlling pain.

I went on a quest to find a physician who specialized in thalamic pain. My neurologist had never had any of his stroke patients suffer from thalamic pain. He himself had no one in particular to recommend, so I went about doing what people do, asking medical people and anybody I saw, "Do you know someone who deals with thalamic pain?" I heard the name of my doctor here at Sloan-Kettering two or three times, and I gave her a call. How I got through to her is a mystery to this day. But I did manage to get through to her, and we had a long conversation. She agreed to see me, and I flew here from Chicago. When I got here, she told me she was loathe to see people with thalamic pain because there was so little she could do for them. I told her I was willing to be a guinea pig, to do anything to the pain so I could function. I was uninterested in being a stay-at-home.

Describe the pain for me.

There are different symptoms, and they appear at different times. One thing that is constant is the burning pain. Just under the surface of the skin, it feels that my arm, my leg, and the left side of my face are on fire. It's pretty much constant, and makes a lot of things difficult to do.

In addition, there's the tight-muscle feeling, the taut arm. It's not phantom pain. After seven or eight hours of that feeling, I'm very tired. Another symptom is constant movement of my left hand. The feelings are much more defined in the arm and hand than in the leg and foot. There is some indication that that is because the leg is weight-bearing and isn't in free fall, whereas the arm is. There are days when my arm just shakes. In order for me to have it not shake, I have to either hold it or put it in my pocket.

Then there's what I'll call the "three-finger pain." It affects the little finger, the middle finger and the ring finger. It feels as if there's a vise wrapped around the three fingers and it's closing in. When that pain starts, it doesn't stop until I go to sleep and wake up the next morning. In fact, all of the pains that I've described, when they occur, never completely go away, even with opioids. They are just reduced to a level where I can manage them and carry on. I am never without some form of pain.

Seventeen years after my stroke, I'm in extreme pain when I wake up in the morning. If I have to be somewhere at nine o'-clock, say, I basically have to get up at five-thirty or six, take some opioids, rest, let them take effect, and then I can get up and shower. I have to leave a couple of hours for this every morning.

How do people respond to your pain? How have your interactions with others changed since you've had this pain?

This is probably for me the most difficult part of the pain. There is a fear that if I complain too much about being in pain, there is a credibility gap with my friends, not because they want to disbelieve me, but because I'm still doing things and out there functioning and yet I say that I'm in a lot of pain. The two things don't match up. I'm always afraid the pain will take over relationships. People ask you how you are, and the answer is fine. But knowing that I have this pain syndrome, good friends and family know that if I say fine, I'm lying. On the other hand, they don't really want a full explanation of the pain I may be having on that particular day because there's nothing they can do to help. So it's a conundrum. If you say fine, they don't believe you. If you tell the truth it could become a barrier to relationships because you become a pain in the ass. They know that if they ask you, you're going to give them an earful.

So although it hasn't affected any of my friendships, the fear that it will is a constant companion for me. I don't want it to be in the way, but it is a major part of who and what I am, so it can't be taken away. I've always said that I didn't want the pain to define me, but seventeen years later, I'm on the cusp of having that happen. That's very disturbing. I find myself always on guard about how much I do or don't talk about the pain. If I spend an evening with people and I haven't talked about the pain, I consider that a victory. If the pain doesn't come up in conversation, I'm thrilled. But if people ask about it, there's little I can do to avoid it.

Does it feel good to talk about it?

Literally, I hate talking about it. However, my good friends tell me that they can see in my face when I'm in pain, and they know it. It becomes "What are you doing?" or "How are you doing?" or "Are you taking pills?" or "Have the pills helped you?"

Let me do a brief aside about the pills for a moment. I take opiates for pain control. That's a difficult issue, because there is an assumption on most people's part that if you take an opiate, you will become an addict—whatever that means. I am dependent upon the opiates that I take. Does that make me an addict? I don't know what an addict is. Because American society is narcotic crazy, when you tell somebody you take an opioid, they look at you like "Oh, my goodness, she's going to become addicted." You can tell that reaction instantly when you first meet somebody. It's part of the societal reaction to opiates. People don't differentiate between the legal and the illegal. There is room in society for legal use of opiates without making a value judgment of the person who is using them. However, since we in America have not been able to differentiate between legal and illegal use, there is a perception problem for those who take them legally. Unfortunately, language is important here. I don't use drugs, I take medication.

I have a friend who runs an agency that reintroduces recovering addicts to society. I can remember her saying to me one day, "What do you mean you're dependent? You're an addict!" That was deadly for me. It was like someone had punched me in the stomach, because I have the same views, thoughts, and prejudices that everyone else in society has. Just because I must take opioids to lessen my pain doesn't mean I'm unaware of the stigmas that come with them. Because of those stigmas, it is only recently, after years, that I have come to take as much as I need, and even so there are days when the medications don't touch the pain, especially the three-finger pain. It's not a dosage issue, but an issue of how the brain on that given day reacts to what it is being fed. Still, I monitor myself so carefully. I'm a much more stringent monitor than my physicians are. They tell me to take as much as I need, but I'm afraid. I don't know what I'm afraid of since I've been given permission, but I know I'm afraid.

You said you don't want your pain to define you. Do you view your pain as something "other" than you? Do you view it as an adversary to be defeated or as a part of you?

Both. It's an adversary I must continually fight in order to function. It's an enormous part of who and what I am. That bothers me. I don't want to be the person in pain. I don't want to be pitied. But people feel badly when you're in pain. It's a natural reaction. Since those in my closest circles know that I'm never out of pain, I have to be careful in my interactions with people.

Does your treatment consist entirely of opioid medications now?

Recently, we've added an anticonvulsant. The problem is it makes me very drowsy. If I'm active, I'm okay, but if I take it when I'm sedentary and doing a repetitive behavior such as typing, I fall asleep right away. So although this new ingredient in the mix does help the pain, I'm in a constant fight against the side effects.

Have you tried taking something to wake you up, to stimulate you?

Unfortunately, I'm medicine sensitive. Things that work one way for other people seem to have opposite effects on me. I originally tried anticonvulsants six years ago, but had drastic problems. Every muscle in my body ached.

Some people portray using opioids as a sort of constant nirvana. Is that your experience?

Certainly not. Opioids are a pain in the neck. Because of the opioids, constipation is my constant companion. I spend my life dealing with it. I eat as much fiber as I can, psyllium husks and so on, but it's a tough battle. Constant constipation gives me urinary problems. I take the medication because it has been legally prescribed to me by a doctor. I'm dependent on it, but I don't go out on the street looking for opioids for recreational purposes, to feel good. When I'm not in a lot of pain, I don't take opioids. They're the last thing on my mind. The problem is that because my body is now dependent on a level of opioids, when I don't take them, I go into a mini withdrawal.

What does that feel like?

I cry, I'm nervous, I get chills, I'm cold. Any or all of the above. That tells me I need to take a small amount, and within twenty minutes I'll be okay. I hate them. I hate being looked at like an addict. I don't even know what that word, what its concept, means. I hate it when people throw words around, when they say, "I'm addicted to painkillers" and then get a lot of media play.

Tell me about the process of procuring your medication.

It's not so easy. Not all doctors will write prescriptions for opioids. If my doctor is on vacation, and I've miscalculated the amount of opioid that I need, I have to find a doctor who will write me a prescription for narcotics. Not only that, but not every pharmacy carries them. The regimen is as follows: I have to figure out how many pills I need for a given period of time. As I get close to running out, I call the pharmacy to make sure the medication is in stock and then tell them that I'm going to have a prescription for x number of pills within the week. Then I call the doctor to make sure that the prescription is written and called in on time.

Have you had difficulties with the pharmacy?

I use only one pharmacy now, and they know me. In the beginning, they filled the prescription, but I perceived some looks of "What is she taking this for?" Over the years my doctor and I have tried a variety of different medications, and whenever that happens I go to the pharmacy and remind them that I have this pain syndrome and explain that this is a new medication we're trying. I feel lucky to have a group of pharmacists now who know me and treat me well.

The juggling act that you're describing, dealing with doctors, pills and pharmacies, sounds very difficult, and it sounds as if you're never really totally in control of your life or your pain.

You hit the nail on the head. In my past life, before the pain struck, I was a control person. Now I feel totally out of control over almost every aspect of my life because I am totally dependent on a whole variety of things in order for me to function at all. I feel the pain least when I'm lying down quietly, without any external stimulus—no television, no radio, nothing. But to me, that's not a life. I want to be a functioning member of society. I want to be active. That's where the problems begin.

Penney Cowan

୧୨

Chronic pain patient Penney Cowan is the founder of the American Chronic Pain Association (ACPA). She and her husband live in Rocklin, California. I interview her there.

Tell me how the ACPA came into existence.

I started the ACPA because I am a person who has pain. My pain started twenty-seven years ago, after the birth of my second child. Before that point I was never sick a day in my life. I was a very active person. During the first six years of pain, I went from doctor to doctor trying to find a solution. It became very clear that the pain was something I was going to have to live with, but nobody told me how to do that.

I was sent to the Cleveland Clinic in Ohio to get a confirmation of the diagnosis. At that point, I met a physician who told me he could help me. I didn't believe him for a second, because I had been told so often that I would have to live with the pain. I agreed to go into the pain-management program to prove to everyone that I was going to fail, that there was nothing anybody could do for me, that the pain was going to consume my life and who I was. I had already lost my identity. Everyone kept telling me—especially my husband—that I could beat it, and I really resented all that. I just wanted to be left alone. When I entered the pain program as a patient, things were so bad I could barely hold a cup of coffee. Seven weeks later I left the pain program a functioning person again, in every sense of the word.

One of the things that struck me while I was in the program was that there were others in chronic pain. During those first six years, I really isolated myself. I thought, in some sense, that my pain was my fault. I really felt a sense of responsibility for not getting better. In the pain program, I found that there were other people like me who were normal in form, because pain doesn't show, but I believed they had pain. So at the end of that time, I was a little bit afraid, because I could manage the pain in a controlled environment, but I didn't know how I would do when I got home and was faced with daily responsibilities. I was also afraid that it was a quick fix, that it would work for a while, but it wouldn't last. So I started a support group in the Pittsburgh area, to let other people know that they are not alone, and to maintain my own wellness.

How did helping other people help you maintain your wellness?

We all need a purpose in life, and for those first six years, pain became my identity. Everything else was taken away from me. Our pain consumes us and becomes us, see? In teaching others what I had learned in the pain program, in reinforcing my basics, I also explored other aspects of managing pain that didn't apply only to me. So it really helped me to research and learn and open myself up. I came to understand chronic pain, pain management, and what it does to our daily lives—what are the issues we really have to face.

My pain affected me in one way. Pain affects others in other ways. So, in listening to them and understanding what their needs were, everything began to develop. Our first manual came out of the first couple of years of groups. Because I needed to give people a foundation, I came up with ten steps. Those ten steps, from patient to person, are really the basis of the organization now.

How were you responsible for your own pain?

When you go to doctors, you expect them to do something. You expect them to give you a pill, to do some kind of surgery or procedure. The end result is either that it all goes well, or the test is negative, meaning there is nothing wrong with you. But when you sit there and look to a physician to fix you, to cure you, to take away your pain, and then you're told that there is no reason for your pain, that there is nothing they can do for your pain, you begin to think you've done something wrong. You figure you didn't follow instructions correctly, or you figure that the problem is simply in your head, that you're imagining things.

I have talked to a lot of people who have had as many as twenty back surgeries, every one of which was a success, and yet there is still pain. So those of us in pain feel that it's our fault—that the pain is because of something we did. Way back when, I even looked to see why I was being punished. I asked God what I did wrong—asked him why I was being singled out for my pain. A lot of people feel that way.

It's a paradox, because we also give responsibility for curing us to physicians. That's part of the contract. We see them as experts who know how to fix us.

One of the problems is that doctors are taught to cure, not to help people manage a pain problem. When you cross over the line to chronic pain, the rules change. What that means is that the person in pain has to become part of the treatment team. They have to accept some of the responsibility. There are certain things we need to do to improve the quality of our lives and reduce our sense of suffering. But physicians were never trained to regard the patient as an equal partner, and they need to be, because we look to them for some things, but they have to look to us to do the things they or their peers are teaching us how to do—relaxation, physical therapy, and so on.

Tell me about your "ten steps."

The ten steps include what I consider the basics. You have to accept the pain, get involved, recognize your priorities, set realistic goals, have a good exercise program, and recognize emotions. Physicians typically don't get into the body/mind link, but we have to understand how those emotions affect our pain. We have to know what our basic rights are—the right to make mistakes, the right to do less than humanly possible, the right to say no and not feel guilty. We have to take what we've learned and go out into the community. Those are the basic steps, but if you look at pain management, you realize that what we are teaching are nothing more than good living skills. Anyone can benefit from what we teach, regardless of whether they have pain or not. Pain has forced us to take a second look at life and how we manage it, and in managing our life, we are also beginning to manage our pain.

It sounds to me as if the ten steps are about becoming more awake. Tell me about the right to do less than humanly possible.

A long time ago I realized that a lot of people with chronic pain tend to be overachievers with low self-esteem. We base who we are on how much we can do. If we work really hard and contribute as much as we can to society, then everyone else is going to tell us we're really great and then we'll feel good about ourselves. Of course, that doesn't work. Rather than taking things slowly, pacing ourselves, we push ourselves and look for acceptance from others. When you have a bad day, you have the right to do less than humanly possible. You don't have to push yourself. Pacing yourself, recognizing your limits and working within them, those are important elements in managing chronic pain. The point is to focus on your abilities, not your disabilities.

So there is a particular personality type associated with the sufferer of chronic pain?

Hopefully, it's not a sufferer of chronic pain. Let's call them people with pain. I hate it when I hear people refer to themselves as chronic pain patients. That's a terrible label. Let's not have that be our identity. We are people with pain. I've had all kinds of people stumbling over that. As far as personality type, I'm certainly one of those A Type people. A long time ago, when they first started looking at chronic pain, they thought they were all blue-collar workers who had chronic pain so they didn't have to go back to work in the coal mines, that sort of thing. Really, it's anyone. It tends to be people who work very hard and have that A Type personality because we don't stop if we get sick. We don't give ourselves enough time to heal. If we have surgery and they tell us to take six months, we take two and say, "Hey, I gotta get back to work." Really, we are pushers, and we create our own problems.

Do you have thoughts about the relationship between pain and suffering?

I believe we have some ability to control the amount of suffering we have. The way I look at it, if we focus on our pain, we're going to suffer a lot. If we can find a way to redirect our attention from our pain onto something we have more control over, we are not going to suffer as much. I tell people to count to twenty-five at the same exact time that they're saying the alphabet. We can't do that. We really have a one-track mind. So if we're thinking about a relaxation technique, if we're imagining how our breath looks as we inhale and it fills our lungs, we cannot also be thinking, at that moment, about how much our back is hurting or our head is pounding. In that way, we can reduce our sense of suffering. It's not always going to work, but it's a good pain-management skill.

Compassion seems to be a pain-management tool for you. Did you find much compassion around you before you found it within yourself?

Probably the most intense passion that I experienced was with my husband. I didn't get that in the first six years from my health care providers. When I got to the pain program, though, I sensed an enormous amount of compassion. People finally understood— not just the people going through the program, but the providers at all levels, from the director to the orderlies—that chronic pain was an invisible disability and that they had to give us encouragement and focus on our well behaviors and ignore our sick behaviors. Reaching out to another person and then having that person reach out to another person is a big part of what keeps me motivated today.

You made what might fairly be called a Freudian slip when talking about your passion for your husband, so let's talk about passion rather than compassion. Do you think passion has a place in pain management?

Earlier I talked about low self-esteem. The passion between my husband and me might have something to do with the fact that he has always been my safe person—the one person in my life whom I could do or say anything around. He always accepts me. He doesn't reject me. He loves me for who I am, not for who other people think I should be. He is my best friend. When you feel really really strongly about something or someone, it really keeps you going. The passionate connection my husband and I share keeps me motivated in our marriage, and the passion I feel for the issues around chronic pain keep me motivated in my work.

Do you think that this is because when the mind is passionately, enthusiastically, or romantically engaged, it cannot simultaneously engage pain?

That's partly true. We choose where our mind is going to go. While I'm working in my office, I'm very focused and I don't think about my pain at all. When I'm with my husband, at any level, whether it be sitting at the dinner table or making love, there is this real sense of connection, like we're one. We've been that way since the day we met.

And that diminishes your pain.

Because it makes me feel better about who I am. Because I am accepted. Because I can just let everything down. That is a part of pain management. Accepting who you are.

So there is a link between the degree of self-esteem and the experience of pain?

Definitely.

What is your medical diagnosis?

I have fibromyalgia. Twenty-seven years ago, it was called fibrocytis, which was kind of a garbage-can diagnosis, and that contributed to my self-doubt about my pain. Even today people don't really understand fibromyalgia, because it isn't something that is black and white. You can't give a blood test for it. You can't do an X ray and see it. It's more a diagnosis of elimination.

The notion of depending on outside diagnosis and validation for what one is feeling inside is a strange one, and yet we do it all the time.

One thing that the ACPA does for people with pain is that we validate them. We don't ask them to defend their pain. We don't ask them to justify it. I believe them. It doesn't matter what the cause of the pain is. None of that matters. Validation is the one thing that people with pain want more than anything else. I don't know how many people have told me "I'd rather have cancer. At least it would be something real." That's really sad, but that's exactly how so many of us feel. We want to be validated. We want someone to believe us. One of the things that the director of my pain program did right away was to tell me that he believed me and that he could help me. Period, end of story.

Do most of the people who come to the ACPA have fibromyalgia, or is it a catchall?

These days it's a catchall. Any kind of pain. I get people who have cancer. It doesn't matter.

They're just looking for that first compassionate step—validation.

That's exactly right. To have someone answer the phone is wonderful to them, and to actually talk to someone who has some understanding is, too. We don't have to talk about their physical symptoms, because in a conversation I can connect with them by knowing what pain does to their lives. I can validate them without putting them in a depressing patient role.

So validation is the first step and connection is the second. Both are elements of compassion.

The individual has to have compassion for themselves in order to reach out. People who call or e-mail or write a letter really have to have some sense of themselves. If this organization had been available to me before I went to the pain program, I don't think I would have believed in myself enough to reach out. People who reach out have this tiny grain of hope in them. They haven't given up, even though they say they have.

A tiny grain of hope that someone will care?

Yes. Someone who will believe them, talk to them, validate them. Then, of course, they also believe that there must be a better quality of life out there for them. Interestingly, a lot of folks are not looking for the pain to be gone, they're just looking to regain some control of their lives.

Stephanie Staker

Stephanie Staker works as a paralegal in Antioch, California. She has suffered from chronic back pain since 1980. The diagnosis is spinal stenosis, facet hypertrophy, and a herniated intervertebral disc at L3 and L4. I interview her sitting outside at a picnic table near her office.

Do you remember the day your pain began?
In 1980, I tripped on my girlfriend's steps and fell. My back was wrenched in the fall, and it has hurt ever since.

Do you remember a time when you did not have pain in your back?
Not in the last twenty years. There have been days when the pain was easier than others, and, of course, days when the pain receded into the background rather than being in the foreground, but never a day when there was no pain at all.

Can you imagine what it might feel like not to have pain now?
Well, yes, I can. If I didn't have the things that were wrong with me today, I could enjoy my grandchildren without limits. I could lift the kids, which I can't do anymore unless I really, really, want to pay for it. I can't even hold my twenty-pound granddaughter unless I'm sitting.

Even though your pain is well controlled?
That's right.

So what you're really talking about is imagining not having the syndromes that lead to your pain?

Having the pain on the back burner is a lot better than having it on the front burner. I don't want to think about it all the time. I don't want it to distract me from things that are more important.

What are some of those things?

God, for one. I'm a born-again Christian. I have been since I was young. Initially, I thought my pain might be a test of my faith. At the time my pain started, I belonged to a church where we were told that if our faith were strong enough, God would heal us. I had experienced some other healings, and I couldn't understand why my pain wasn't being healed. I got very depressed about it. Finally, I came to a point of acceptance. Like Paul with the thorn in his side, I figure this is my thorn.

Did you ever get angry with God?

For a time I did. That's a stage in any grief process. For a while, when I couldn't do things that I used to do, things that I wanted to do, I was angry at myself and I was angry at Him.

Grieving is usually associated with loss. What did you feel you had lost?

I had lost freedom—the freedom to do things to which I never gave a second thought—things that are now very costly in terms of the pain I feel later if I do them. That continues today. As my back degenerates, I'm finding that there are more things I have to be careful of. I have to be very aware of body mechanics all the time. As a kid, of course, I never thought about those things at all.

Did you feel guilty in some way for being angry with God, or feel that He was judging you?

I absolutely did feel guilty. I felt that somehow my faith wasn't good enough, that somehow I didn't believe enough. I still don't know the answer to how one generates more faith, enough belief in order to be healed. I have a peace about it now, though. That's the only word I can use about it. Peace.

You mentioned that you experienced other healings in your church.
That's right. I had cervical dysplasia. Precancerous cells in the uterus. I was having to have treatment for it every month, and was having to have a monthly Pap smear looking for abnormal cells. Then one day I went forward for a prayer, and I never had an abnormal Pap smear from that time on. That was in 1981.

When you said you "went forward for a prayer," what did you mean, exactly?
I went forward and had other people pray for me. I prayed with them, too. Then a couple or three weeks later, I went to my next appointment, and the test was negative. It was negative a month later, too, and that was when the specialist turned me over to my regular family doctor, who monitored me on a sixth month basis, and then yearly.

Were the pain medications you initially received helpful?
They were, but then my body got used to them and they didn't work as well anymore. I didn't understand what "drug tolerance" meant back then. Nobody explained that to me, and I didn't know that was what was going on. I thought that there was something wrong with me when I needed to increase my dose.

Did you worry that your condition was deteriorating?
Of course I did, but I was in denial. I didn't want to accept that it might be getting worse. I told myself it was the same, and I was just becoming a whiner. I didn't have the support of my then spouse. He said that I was a complainer, that I always said there was something wrong with me. It's funny, because I look at my-

self now and I don't think I'm a complainer at all. My family doctor now worries because he thinks I'm too stoic.

Where did you learn to be stoic?

It might be an issue of family upbringing. I can remember as a child when I'd have a headache and tell my mother. She would say, "You can't have a headache. You're too young." I would be dismissed, as it were. The unspoken half of that was, "Be quiet, don't talk about it, don't tell *me* about it." The biggest thing for me, at the time, was that if my mother said I couldn't be having a headache, and I was, then there must be something wrong with my sense of reality. It must be something I was making up. Being stoic started at an early age for me, and it included things beyond physical pain. Fear, for example. I couldn't be afraid. That wasn't an acceptable emotion for me. Of course, you have to understand, my mother was crippled when she was a child. From the time she was eighteen months old, she had polio. She dealt with a lot of physical pain herself.

So she didn't want to hear too much complaining?

That's correct. She was very much the stoic herself.

And where do you suppose she got that?

Same place I got it. Family culture. She came from a very unhappy family. Her father was an alcoholic, and her mother died when she was fifteen. Her mother was an Orthodox Jew, and her father was an Irish Catholic. There was religious diversity, but there was also animosity between the two families. The funny thing is, I, myself, identify with both religions now.

My grandmother died from an abortion. That was before abortions were legal. My grandfather abandoned my mother—and her sister, my aunt—after that. He left them in the care of my great-grandmother. So there were some strong dynamics going on in my mother's life, some real suffering that she had to put up with. Maybe this wasn't so much a religious thing for her, but a result of her experience. She had a hard time.

How did the people in your adult life respond to your pain when it began?

Initially, my children had the same reaction as their father. They said I was a complainer. My son doesn't say that kind of thing any more. Age brings compassion. Of course, now, my son sees me function. He's an attorney, and I work in the law office with him. It was coming to work with me when I was a paralegal and he was just a kid that got him interested in law. So he sees me do things as well as I can. He has more respect for that now. At the time that my chronic pain started, I had a lot of friends, born-again Christians, who chided me, who said I didn't believe strongly enough. That added to my guilt. They tried to say that if I had had greater faith, I wouldn't have had the pain.

So God looks around and gives pain to those who lack faith?

I suppose it all boils down to that. About a year after my chronic back pain started, I began having female problems. Nothing to do with my cervix, but I had to have a hysterectomy. This one particular friend, who, at that time, was my best friend, said that I had turned to the Devil, to Satan, because I opted to have a hysterectomy. She thought I should have had more faith, and that God would have healed me if I did, and that having a medical failure was a sign of my religious weakness, my failure.

Taking pain medications might fall into the same category, then, as having surgery?

That's right. But I'm on opioid analgesics now, and I have to tell you, I don't have any issues with lack of faith or that kind of guilt any longer.

What new model do you have that gives you peace about all that?

For one thing, I've educated myself. I didn't even know that there was such a phenomenon, such a syndrome, as chronic pain. I've learned to accept that I have it, and I've gone through the grieving process I talked about earlier. I want a life. I deserve to be able to function in the world, with my family and friends, and my job. The way that I do that is by taking medication. Even if I didn't have back problems, I know that as time goes on that our bodies don't work the same. That's unfortunate, but it's true. I have come a long way in my own thinking about acceptance, about the person I am today. That includes taking medications to minimize my pain and give me a life, to allow me to sleep, to enjoy my husband, my kids, my grandchildren, particularly. I remarried four years ago, by the way.

How long has your pain been well controlled?

For about a year and a half. Out of twenty years in pain, I spent eighteen and a half suffering and trying a succession of specialists and modalities. At first I was prescribed antiinflammatory drugs that gave me lots of side effects. They're very hard on the liver and the kidneys. The heart too, in some cases. Actually, they gave me gastroesophageal reflux disease. And I was given a lot of steroid injections, which, as it turns out, have actually led to more problems with my back. I have few side effects with opioid medications, except constipation, which is serious, and I have to deal with that.

Why do you figure good pain control took so long?

For one thing, not all physicians are equally knowledgeable or equally competent. Also, prejudices about addiction get in the way. The war on drugs, which started in the 1960s, has made physicians afraid of regulatory agencies, of state medical boards, of the DEA. They're afraid of having their licenses taken away. It happens all over the United States, and it's really sad. Doctors just giving patients what they need get in trouble. My own pain doctor has been under investigation by the state attorney general. He has a good attorney himself, and he's managed to keep them at bay, but it's terrible. The bottom line is that it is easier for these agencies to hassle the physicians than it is to go get the drug dealer. There's a paper trail with doctors. They know where the doctors are.

As voters, we have sent the message that we have to do something about drugs on the street. I agree with that, but it's not so simple. Unfortunately, there are people who get drugs from a compassionate doctor and then turn around and sell them. But a good pain-management doctor takes the time to check out his patients. He finds out if they're abusers; he assesses them medically; he has to have a referral and some records, with a diagnosis that validates the pain. Of course, that doesn't mean that a few bad apples can't get through the system.

I've learned about a lot of this through an Internet pain group. I trade e-mails with other sufferers. I learn about the situation, and it's pretty eye-opening. That's where I realized the difference between tolerance and addiction. Even my own family doctor didn't know about that. I brough her the printed Web page and showed it to her. There are some doctors who really like you to be an informed patient, who like you to do research and stuff, and there are others who feel very threatened by it. I like a doctor I can work with. I like to be an active partner in managing my own health. I'm the kind of person who is at peace if I know what's going on.

Our society needs to know about the difference between tolerance and addiction, and they need to know that there is such a thing as chronic pain syndrome. I didn't know it, and I was a chronic pain sufferer! If I am one and I don't know it, there is something wrong with the way we're getting out the word.

Susan Shinagawa

❧

Susan Shinagawa lives near San Diego, California, with her husband and her two dogs. She is a third-generation Japanese American (sansei) and is forty-four years old. I interview her on a warm, late-summer day, in her backyard, under an umbrella.

You have had some serious medical problems.

Well, I'm a two-time primary, one-time recurrent breast cancer survivor. In 1991, I had my first primary breast cancer. I had a modified radical mastectomy and axillary node dissection, followed up by eight cycles of adjuvent chemotherapy. I did fine until November of 1996, when I started exhibiting symptoms of left-sided weakness and pain, chronic nausea, headaches and was eventually diagnosed in January of 1997 with recurrent breast cancer present in my cerebral spinal fluid. That condition is called carcinomatous meningitis—CM for short. I was treated with intrathecal chemotherapy, meaning chemotherapy delivered directly to my cerebral spinal fluid through my brain. I also had received radiation to my lumbar spine.

In July 1997 I finished my chemo and started going to the pain clinic at the UCSD Medical Center for the chronic lumbar pain that was the legacy of my recurrence. In January 2001, a second primary cancer on the left breast was found by a mammogram. In February, I had a second mastectomy, and a sentinel node biopsy, and because it was an early stage breast cancer and because I was still getting all kinds of drugs for my pain, I decided not to have any adjuvant chemotherapy for that cancer.

Tell me about the pain you have now.

It sucks. I don't know what else to say about it. It's in my lumbar spine, which is where it has always been. On the little wonderful 1 to 10 pain scales they give you, my baseline is about a 6.5. I have a continuous infusion pump implanted in my abdomen, and that gives me intrathecal opioid narcotics every day, 24 hours a day. That and opioid patches that I wear get me to about a 5.0. Sometimes I get down below 4.0, but I would say that for every two good days, days where the pain is a 4.0 or 5.0, I have one day that is kind of so-so, where the pain is at my baseline, and one and a half days on which the pain gets up to 7.5 or 8.0 and I can't even get out of bed.

In consultation with my pain doc, I've decided to change my pain regimen so that I can enroll in two clinical trials. The first involves an in-depth analysis of my cerebrospinal fluid and allows me control over my pump for an additional dose every eight hours if I need it. Currently, I have no control over my dose other than to show up at the clinic and ask for an increase, which I do whenever I'm in town. I know that studies show that post-surgical patients with similar control during hospitalization use less pain meds than their control counterparts—those who have to ask a nurse for pain meds. I suppose this study may be looking for similar results. I, on the other hand, am looking for increased pain control—period. I've had a rough last week and just can't afford the "down time" resulting from these periods of incapacitating pain.

When the pump runs out, how do they recharge it?

The pump is like a hockey puck. It has a little rubber flange in it. When I need a refill, they stick a needle through my skin and into the flange and fill it up. They program my dosage on a computer, then let that computer talk to the one in the pump. The computer tells me when my next pump alarm date will be, which is two days before the drug will be used up, and then I know when to schedule my next appointment. So I go back to have a refill about every six or eight weeks.

How long does the pump battery last?

About five years. The computer lets us know when the battery is running low, and then they have to take the pump out surgically and put a new one in and at the same time put a new catheter from the pump to the intrathecal space in my spinal cord.

Do you work?

I went on sick leave in December 1996, when I first got the pain and left side weakness. Then, in January I went on the Family Medical Leave Act for three months, and then in March of 1997 I went on medical disability. The pain hurts a lot more when I'm not busy, and I drive myself crazy if I don't do something, so I volunteer as a cancer advocate and, more recently, as a pain advocate. I work with a number of different nonprofit organizations—mostly national, some state, a couple local—that deal with pain and cancer, primarily in minority and medically underserved populations, which is a euphemism for poor.

What led you to advocacy work?

The fact that there's a need for it. You know, everybody says that you don't know what it's like to have cancer until you have cancer. Well it's that way for pain too. You *really* don't know what it's like to have pain until you have pain. For the longest time, people thought I was making it up, or that my pain was all in my head. Not all the doctors, but some of the doctors thought that, and so did people in my extended family, which was very aggravating.

Part of the advocacy work has also been selfish. I had never realized that when you're in a wheelchair, people don't see you. I travel for some of the volunteer work, and I'm amazed by some of the things that happen to me. If you're walking with a cane and clearly in pain, for example, people won't open a heavy door for you or give you their seat.

My doctor at the pain clinic tells me how frustrating it is to have daily arguments with other physicians about prescribing adequate narcotic analgesia for their patients. Even some doctors, who should know better, think that their patients are going to become drug addicts. It's ridiculous.

How could anyone, much less a family member, disbelieve that you would have pain from metastatic disease?

I am a third-generation Japanese American, a *sansei*. Even though I am third generation, there are still some things about me that are very Japanese. I was brought up in a house that had a lot of Japanese cultural nuances. One of the things that I grew up learning was this thing called *gaman*. To gaman means not to burden others with your problems, in this case not to complain about my pain. Basically, you're supposed to be stoic—to keep your problems to yourself. You're not supposed to complain about pain, and you're not supposed to burden other people with your pain and your problems.

I learned to gaman very well. When I was in high school, I was waterskiiing and I fell and hit my tailbone really hard on the ski. It was such a bad fall that for a little while I was paralyzed in the water. I mean, I couldn't move. A little while later, I started having really bad pain in my tailbone. I didn't want anyone to touch me, because it hurt so bad. My dad wanted to call an ambulance. Now I also grew up really conscious of money, and how much things cost, and I didn't really have a concept of insurance at the time and I didn't want him to have to pay for the ambulance, so I sucked it and I got in the car and we went to the emergency room and I did what I was supposed to do, which was sit there and be quiet, even though I had tears in my eyes. So we were put in this room, where we had to sit for two hours. Finally my dad said "Susan, I don't want you to gaman anymore. I want you to make noise. I want them to know you're in pain." He had to tell me not to gaman. That was the only time he ever told me that.

So that's how I deal with my pain. I gaman a lot. It's not something I think about, it's just what I do—how I am. My husband and his family are not Japanese. They're not familiar with the concept of gaman. Most of the time, I don't complain about my pain. I'm a person who has been very independent and is very aggressive and very assertive and takes care of things. If something has to be done I want to take care of it myself, even if it hurts to do so. So the reason people don't think I have pain—I don't really know, I'm just assuming here—is that I don't complain about it. Also, I will force myself to do things unless I'm having one of those really bad days and I'm in bed and can't get out. If I'm not having one of those days, I'm out trying to do what I can, whatever needs to be done. That's just how I am. That's just how I've always been. So I guess if people think that I'm the way that I've always been, then I must not really have pain.

What have you learned from your advocacy work?
The most common thing is that other folks think you're a drug addict if you're taking narcotics, and why on earth would you let someone give you those drugs. Another thing is the whole physical thing. Unless you're screaming and bleeding, people don't show you compassion, especially if you're young. Maybe they think you just sprained your ankle. That's what people always ask me when I walk with a cane when traveling. "What did you do to

your leg, what did you do to your leg?" They always want to know what I did to my leg, but nobody ever thinks that it's anything major.

How do you answer the question?

It depends, and frankly I don't know what makes me answer one way or the other. Sometimes I just tell them that my back hurts. Sometimes I tell them I've had cancer in my spine. That kind of stops the conversation right there. If I don't want to say anything else, that's what I say. Sometimes, of course, I just say that because I need to tell the truth. I have actually asked people at the airport if I could sit in a seat next to them and had them say, "Oh, my wife's going to sit there," or "Oh, my husband is going to sit there" or "No, I need that seat for my bag." I've actually had someone tell me that I couldn't sit down. It's amazing. Once I actually got stuck in a bathroom because I didn't have the strength to open the door. I had to wait for someone to come and open the door for me. Things like that are frustrating, and at times, aggravating.

Do you think that this is because you look young and relatively healthy, or because people are genuinely compassionless?

I don't know what people are thinking. Most of the time I look okay, sometimes I look pretty bad. When I'm traveling, I try not to look sick. I try to look normal. It's just that they don't realize what's going on. Of course there are people who genuinely lack compassion, but I like to think they are the minority. I do run into people who are definitely clueless. And then there are people who are incredibly kind and really go out of their way to be helpful.

You just mentioned looking normal. Do you remember what normal feels like? Do you remember what it is like not to have great pain?

That's a good question. (*crying*) Yes, I do remember what it feels like, and I keep thinking I'm going to get back there. I still believe that I will. The year before I got sick, meaning the year before I had this back pain, I went snow skiing for the first time. I was awesome. I was so cool at it! I was ready to go to the Olympics the next day. I kept falling down, but by the end of the day I could get up faster than anyone else because I had fallen so many times and I had to learn to get up by myself. But I loved it. And then, you know, I wanted to go skiing again the next winter, but that's when I got sick.

I still want to go skiing. I used to be a rock climber. We used to go hiking a lot. We used to go to Yosemite every year and hike. Every year. We didn't just go drive around the valleys the way some people do. We liked to get out there, to go camping and backpacking. I bought a mountain bike when I met my husband. We used to go riding every weekend. Whenever we went on vacation we took our bikes. We used to have so much fun! I don't get to do all those fun things anymore. I spend almost all of my time inside now. I spend a lot of time at home because I can't drive anymore. I haven't driven in four years because the drugs I take make me tired and I fall asleep a lot without knowing it. Also, I can't turn around and check my blind spot, so it's a little scary driving when you don't feel like you have full control.

I recently met with a breast surgeon to discuss bilateral breast reconstruction. The best option, from my perspective, is a latissimus translap in which they would move the large muscles from my back to the chest wall and then augment that with saline implants. There are obviously pros and cons to this and other surgical options, but the most significant point against this option is that I won't be able to snow ski again, because I won't have the muscles needed to work the poles, specifically to pick my butt off the ground when I fall down! It's a ten-hour surgery. I'm still in the thinking process.

Does your back hurt less when you're having fun?

I don't think fun has a whole lot to do with it. I try to distract myself from the pain a lot. The advocacy work helps. I'm either sitting at the computer, which I can't do for very long, or I'm out and about. It takes me a long time to do things I used to be able to whip out in half an hour. My brain is slower, and my body doesn't like to stay still.

This summer, my dad was really sick and so I went and lived with my folks for the summer. I took care of my dad while he was in the hospital for almost two months. I basically was his nurse, other than giving him drugs. He recovered, although he's now back in the hospital. We didn't think he was going to make it through the summer. The whole time I was up there, I missed going to my appointments at the pain clinic. I came back to San Diego once, because I had to have my pump refilled. If you don't get your pump refilled, you go through withdrawal. I made the mistake of doing that the first time. I didn't know that you have to get it refilled right away, and I went through withdrawal. I didn't want to do that again, so I flew home to get my pump refilled on time. Taking care of my dad when I thought he was going to die was not fun at all, but it was a distraction. So when I can get distracted, I don't feel the pain so much. It's always there, and I'm always slow and it always affects me, but it doesn't feel so bad.

Do you consider yourself addicted to narcotics?

No, I don't. For one thing, for the dose of narcotics I take, if I was addicted to them, they should be making me high or something, and they're not. I've never once felt like I was high. What they do to me is to make me feel tired. Sometimes, when I'm getting used to a new drug, my speech is slurred. My speech is always much, much slower than it used to be. That's the thing that I feel the most—that my brain doesn't work the way it used to work, the way that I want it to work. I don't feel like I'm on drugs. The only thing they do for me is to help make my life bearable.

Tell me about the advocacy work itself.

A lot of it is public speaking, meeting with lawmakers, policymakers, public policy people. Sometimes it involves writing reports. There are a lot of educational activities for the public, and for the medical community and researchers.

What is the theme of the work?

A lot of my pain advocacy is very similar to my cancer advocacy. It's focused on the diagnosis and treatment of pain, just like the diagnosis and treatment of cancer, in minority and medically underserved populations. For the big wide world with health insurance and access to medical care, it's not optimal, but if you're a minority, if you have a low literacy level, don't speak English, or are poor, it's a whole other ball game. A lot of studies show that minorities are less often taken seriously about their pain and are undertreated. Medication is expensive. If I myself didn't have my insurance, there would be no way I could afford the meds I need, and there are a lot of folks that can't. That's not right.

I personally believe that everybody who lives in the United States, the richest country in the world, ought to have access to the medical system whenever they need it. A lot of folks don't. Even in the best case scenario, if you're like me, if you have insurance and you know people in the medical field, things don't work well. It took my pain physician two years of writing letters to get my insurance company to approve compounding my pump dose. At the dosage that they approved, I would have had to make the five-hour trip to my clinic *every week* to have the pump refilled. The system sucks. Things need to be better.

Matthew Rudes

~

Matthew Rudes is a fifteen-year-old boy who suffers from spontaneous infantile Marfan syndrome, a rare and devastating form of connective tissue disease, and one that is often fatal at birth. He lives in Los Angeles's San Fernando Valley with his mother, father, and brother. He is confined to a wheelchair. I interview him at his home.

Tell me about Marfan syndrome.

Marfan syndrome affects all the connective tissues in the body. That means it affects everything in the body except the brain. I feel I'm pretty intelligent, and that's really the only thing that Marfan syndrome hasn't affected. I also have a severe chronic pain syndrome, and most of the life I can remember has been filled with pain and surgery.

Can you give me some details about the pain you experience?

Most Marfan people don't have the severity of pain I do. My chronic pain started at age eight or nine. I had this sudden, infuriating back pain one day, and although it was undiagnosed, it kept getting worse and worse. Basically, the pain has changed my life. Everything has to work around it. I never know when it will spring up. I never know when I'll have to go home from school, or leave a movie.

So the pain comes on suddenly and without warning?

Yes. For years I would just literally blank out. It was like I was having a seizure. I could see and hear everything, but I couldn't respond. Sometimes I would go into a state of paralysis, where I just couldn't move. There was one episode where I was in the bathtub when that happened. I would have extreme burning sensations up and down my spine that would last for maybe fifteen or twenty seconds. I would scream and scream in pain. Different things like that would happen.

Tell me about the experience of blanking out.

I felt that I was just in a big black nothingness. I was just there and I could hear everybody and I wanted to respond but my body, my mouth, just wouldn't work until the seizure or whatever you want to call it stopped.

Did you feel pain in that big black nothingness?

No, there wasn't really any sensation. I could usually hear what was going on around me, but I didn't have pain.

And convulsions?

Probably it wasn't exactly a seizure. It was really just a blackout. My head would fall onto my shoulder. There were times when I would move like crazy though, when the electric pains started running up and down my spine. The pain was so horrendous that I would lose control of my body and start flailing about wherever I was. My mother couldn't even stop me. If I was in bed, she used seatbelts that she attached to the bed to strap me down so that I would not be injured further.

Tell me about your surgeries.

I've had two life-saving heart surgeries. My ascending aorta and aortic valve have been replaced twice, and my mitral valve has been repaired. I've had two major back surgeries recently, one spinal fusion to try and help the back pain I've been having and another to remove part of the rods that were placed in my back earlier, because they were causing me pain. When I was very young, I had different ankle and leg surgeries to help me try and walk. Unfortunately they only helped me walk for a short period of time. I've had several eye surgeries, and I've had my gallbladder removed. Overall, I've had thirteen surgeries. I've also been in the hospital quite a few times for pain. At the beginning they used to tell me that nothing was there.

Do you mean they couldn't find a cause for your pain?

A little of both. They felt I was faking pain to get attention. They would do scans and X rays and other tests, and they would come up negative. They then thought it was pretty clear I was faking it.

How did that make you feel?

It made me really *angry*. Sad, too, because I just slip through the cracks of the medical system. If the first or second test didn't reveal something, they left it at that. That affected my life. Most of the seventh, eighth and ninth grades I wasn't there because I had to be home schooled because of my pain episodes. Their rush to a conclusion really screwed up my life, and that makes me really mad, not only for myself, but for other people like me.

I'm one of the longest-lived people with my particular condition, so to some extent my doctors are learning right along with me. Up and down my spine there are little outpocketings of the spinal cord. Nothing can be done to remove them. Most Marfan people have at least one of these pockets at the base of the spine, but I have many. These pockets are even at the back of my eyes. It's possible they press on spinal nerves, which cause me pain, but there's no way to know if that's exactly the cause of my pain.

Is your pain under better control now?

There were literally *years* when our pain was not under control, when we were in agony. Those years of not knowing whether I would lose consciousness the next second, that time when the doctors wouldn't believe me, that was a time when my life was basically *nothing*. If my doctors would have helped our pain at that time, I'm sure I wouldn't need as much medication as I do now. I'm sure I'm worse because of the way they neglected me. I go to a pain specialist now, and that's what he has conveyed to me. I don't think other people want to admit that, because it would mean that they did something wrong. Now I see my pain doctor weekly, and we work together to establish a regimen to deal with our pain, to raise or lower the medication as needed.

Do you tolerate your pain medicines well?

I take opioid analgesics, and they don't have any side effects that I'm aware of, other than slowing me down mentally a little bit. If I went off them I would probably be in severe pain. I mean I could probably write equations about how to get to Saturn, but I'd be screaming, too. The pain medication doses are adjusted up and down so that I can find that place where I can think and act on my own.

How is your relationship with your pain doctor?

He was the first doctor who thought I wasn't faking it. We don't really have a patient/doctor relationship. We're more like friends. He looks after us and we help him in any way possible, although he really does most of the helping. Since everything that happens to me is basically new and mysterious, he helps us try to solve them. He makes sure that when I'm hospitalized, I receive the best care and medications. He writes notes in as basic English as possible to make clear to any doctors or hospital staff that I need as much medication to relieve any pain that can be relieved.

You've been using the words "I" and "me", along with "we" and "us", when referring to your symptoms and experiences. Why is that?

I meant me and my mother. My mother is always there for me.

My whole life. So I feel that my pain is hers also, because she has to take care of me when I have these episodes. I say "our pain" because we're connected. Everything that happens to me, happens to her. Everywhere I am, she's basically there too, or just a phone call away.

When you require homeschooling, does your mother teach you?
A teacher comes over from the school and he teaches me, although my mother helps to motivate me.

Do you do well in school?
I do extremely well. I have a 4.0 grade average in tenth grade. Honors. After I sleep a couple of hours just so I can get up out of my wheelchair, I work every night until ten or eleven o'clock so I can get good grades and go to college and have a career.

Are your teachers sympathetic to your plight?
I have great teachers now. They don't treat me like some poor kid in a wheelchair. They don't mind that I miss assignments sometimes of course, or have to turn them in late or do other things to get the credit, but they don't make excuses for me. They expect a lot from me, and they push me to do my best because I can. They don't treat me like I'm just a cripple or a vegetable who is just going through school because the law says I have to. I think they enjoy having me in class.

How do your peers react to your pain?
Most of the kids at school don't know the full extent of my pain. I may gloat about how many surgeries I've had, about having had my heart valves replaced, but they don't really understand that after school I have to sleep for two hours because I'm so exhausted by the pain. They think that I'm just a kid in a wheelchair. They don't think I'm faking, but they don't understand the level at which I live.

I'm interested in the word "gloat." Does it mean that you have some sat-isfaction of having had surgeries? Does it feel like proof of how bad you really feel?

I don't think it's that. I think it's that I'm proud of being one of three people suffering from such a severe syndrome and still alive. Sharing a tiny bit of that with the people around me helps them understand that I'm not just a person without working legs. It's so much more. I want them to have a small taste of every-thing that's physically wrong.

I noticed a lot of books in your bedroom. What do you like to read most?

Mystery, adventure, sci-fi. Anything that I can benefit and learn from, get someone else's viewpoint, I'll read and love.

Do you spend much time on the computer? Do you play computer games?

I do play computer games. Console games, too, like on the PlayStation and the PlayStation 2. I like the usual Tomb Raider blast 'em, shoot 'em games, and role-playing games, which re-quire thinking. I also like strategy games. In role-playing games you have to control a cast of characters to save the world. That feeling, when you beat the game feels really good—when you beat all those puzzles and you finally get to the end.

There's great satisfaction in saving the world.

Kenneth Anbender, Ph.D.

ಲಿ⊚

A clinical psychologist by training, Kenneth Anbender is the founder and president of Contegrity, Inc., a personal-training organization that has helped thousands of people—in both a private and a corporate setting—find meaning and harmony in their lives. I interview Dr. Anbender in South Florida.

I understand that you have experienced chronic physical pain.

On July 20, 1990, I was poisoned while running a program for about 850 people in Acapulco, Mexico. I didn't know that was what happened. I figured that even though I was at a "five-diamond" hotel, something just got through and I got sick. The poisoning was the beginning of a long slide downhill. Antibiotics didn't help the stomach and lung problems, the pain, the night sweats, nausea, the coughs and other flu-like symptoms. My vitality diminished, my pleasure in life lessened, everything became a battle. In trying to recover and in trying to solve the mystery of what had happened to me, I was initiated into a new world of communicating with doctors.

Did you get depressed?

I had an inspiring job where people counted on me to be upbeat. I was still working with people deeply, but I felt that my mood was under attack, that I was sapped. I had chronic fatigue syndrome, but I didn't know that at the time. This was 1990, and the diagnosis, the syndrome, was still unrecognized by the Centers for Disease Control. One thing that has emerged consistently about the disease is that you may feel way worse than you look, so I looked to doctors like I was in decent shape. But I knew that I was only a fifth of the human being I was before Mexico. I was 80-percent diminished.

Did you have trouble convincing your doctors you felt poorly?
I had an illness that doctors at that time were not sure was an illness. They didn't have much sense of what the patient's inner experience was—what level of pain, of sleep difficulty, of thinking difficulty, brain difficulties, mood distortions went with the package. I considered myself an insightful, clear-thinking, intelligent person who needed a lot of power to do their daily work. This was a time when I had taken over a number of people's jobs and was doing all of them as a test of my communication ability and my power. I go in to talk to a doctor, and, in the state I was in, I felt almost the opposite. I felt like a whiner, a complainer. I didn't look as bad as I felt, and, in order to counter that appearance, I had to say things like "Look, you don't understand. I have a high pain threshold, and it hurts just to sit here."

Did you feel you were being judged?
It had less to do with being judged than being validated. Doctors don't have much room to say "I don't know, but let's find out. Let me refer you to someone who specializes in fatigue or pain." It's amazing how many doctors I've seen who would rather experiment on you—and they get paid to do so—than send you to someone who knows more about your problem. They are willing to let you suffer through it while they experiment diagnostically. Two doctors failed to correctly diagnose what was going on, and while I loved to work and kept going for eight or nine months,

my condition deteriorated and I was able to work fewer and fewer hours per week. My blood pressure went from 110 over 60 to 180 over 120, which led to an essential hypertension diagnosis based on the hard numbers. The doctors could see only what the numbers showed. I literally grabbed one doctor by the lapels—and remember, communication is my field—and said "You don't get it. I can't function. I'm so tired it hurts. Sleep doesn't help. I get up as tired as I go to bed. My body aches in twenty places. Something is going on!"

Finally, a third doctor made the correct diagnosis, but switching doctors is not so easy. You have a folder an inch thick of tests and results. You're tired, you have no memory. Your body aches and you're exasperated. Pain and fatigue make life difficult. The idea of starting all over again to bring a doctor up to speed is overwhelming. You've climbed this mountain with your doctor and then you realize they're not going to the top with you. You have to get down off the mountain and climb another one. It's a horrifying prospect.

Maybe what we're really talking about here is the general difficulty in communicating the invisible.

You're talking to someone who has spent the last thirty years talking to people about the invisible. I'm quite comfortable with that process, but it is difficult to do when there isn't much trust or interest. I didn't go to doctors to tell them my story but to be returned to health—to have a partner in that pursuit who knows more about bodies than I do, because bodies are not my field. I would say to them, "Look, I have some weird symptoms, and they're for real. I'm not a nut. I'm a clinical psychologist. I know how to assess nuts, and I'm not one. Now I'm looking for a partner to help me fix my body." If the doctor were to respond up front, "Look, I'm going to trust only what I see and what has been written up well. Don't expect me to cover any new ground.

Now, would you like to work together?" I would say no and go someplace else. The tricky thing is that's not what people say.

In defense of doctors, I'd say that both the doctor and the patient have something at risk when it comes to trusting each other.

What's at risk is how things are likely to go. I told my doctors that I was hypersensitive to all kinds of medications, yet every doctor gave me a dosage that knocked me for a loop and took a long time to come back from. Every doctor thought they knew better and they gave me too much. I was betting on their interpretation of what I needed to feel better, to heal, to be free of pain. If the doctor risked anything it was his pride.

You say you've made a career out of communicating the invisible. Would you give me an example?

I spent fifteen years working with people to transform the quality of their lives—who they are, what that life is about, how to live well, and, in the last ten years, what fulfills a human life. These things are very value based. They're very much about relationships with others, and with life itself, with the transcendent. You can't just point to these things. They come out of communicating. They're not obvious. I can't really get results with too much clinical dispassion. I have to listen to hear what's unique to the person, what's of real concern to them, what their strengths, depth, and talents are and how to tap them. Ultimately, however, people have to drive their own transformation and healing. They have to see it themselves, you can't see it for them, you can't tell them about the process, you can't force it. It can be assisted, of course, but the healing has to happen from within.

Do you think some doctors make the same decision about relieving physical pain?

If there is pain that moves somebody along in the right direction, I don't mind leaving it there. If there is an amount of pain beyond that, pain that suppresses rather than focuses, something to bear up under rather than something with a creative force, then I don't see any value to it. People can make a lesson out of just about anything, but I don't see value in suffering the pain, the brain fog, the sleep deprivation of chronic fatigue syndrome.

Of course, the distinction between physical and emotional pain is an intellectual construct. The death of a child or the end of a long-term relationship can make a person double over just as surely as a blow to the belly. The biological mechanism may be different, but the effect may be similar.

People are way more resilient about emotional pain than physical pain. I have seen an insight take someone from the depths of despair to a state of freedom even when nothing about the circumstances of life has changed. I haven't seen that so much in physical pain. Ghandi wrote a guide to health. He started it out with two interesting points. The first thing he said was, if you don't get any air you'll die in minutes; if you don't get any water you'll die in days; if you don't get any food you'll die in weeks. Those are the priorities. If you want to talk about health, start with air—which we never talk about—breathing well and quality of air. Then talk about the quality of water and, then, food. It makes perfect sense. Ghandi had that kind of sensibility. Turning the pyramid upside down.

After that, Ghandi goes on a tirade against aspirin and digestive aids. He said he's totally against them, says people eat too much. An alarm goes off. They feel crummy. They take an antacid, and it shuts off the alarm. They continue to keep eating too much. And they drink too much. Then, they get a headache. They take an aspirin. They keep eating and drinking too much, and they wonder why their health gets trashed later on." He says, we're shutting off the alarm. People can eat and drink less if it sets off an alarm. So when something can be done, and I have to figure that up until the end stages of conditions, or in sudden trauma, it always can—I'm more of a fan of fixing what made the alarm go off. Most conditions develop slowly. If it is possible to manage the pain by doing something about its cause, then I favor that. If it gets too far, if the body is trashed, then, of course, pain should be relieved.

So when you went to the doctor suffering from chronic fatigue syndrome, you were looking for the cause of the alarm.

I figured something wasn't working. It read out as pain, and fifty other things, and I wanted to know what the alarm signified and what I could do about it.

Do you think most patients want the alarm turned off, or do they want to know what it's telling them?

I think both, and that might be the first diagnostic category to come up with. It may even be more important than what specific condition they have. In the arenas I'm familiar with, if I hear that someone wants the alarm turned off, I won't do it. Sometimes I can't do it.

If pain is a warning bell, who do you suppose put it there?

There is pain in life. It is hard to imagine going through life without it. But what's fascinating is that there is beauty possible, there is fulfilment possible, and sometimes that even comes through pain or out of pain. It would be interesting if doctors would talk about managing pain in terms of producing beauty, in terms of alleviating pain to allow patients the time to create beauty, or leaving some pain in place to allow people to "evolve toward beauty."

So if you taught a medical school course, what might your pain-management credo be?

Medicine is about compassion. If you attempt to heal without compassion, you may be doing as much damage as good. I suppose my credo would be: "Act compassionately in a way that fulfills life."

Deborah Hunter

Deborah Hunter is thirty-eight years old. She studied marketing management at Long Island University, served in the military, and now serves as a corrections officer at Riker's Island, a large facility in the New York City prison system. She has had debilitating headaches since she was a child. I interview her at her doctor's office on Long Island.

Tell me about your headaches.

I've had them since I was a child. As I've gotten older, the pain has gotten worse, and has lasted a lot longer. I've gone from doctor to doctor over the years, from childhood to high school to college. To this point, nobody has found the cause of the problem or found medicines to cure me or even keep the pain down more than a little. I use over-the-counter products, or just deal with the pain, but often I end up in the emergency room.

How often do you get these headaches?

It's normal for me to have a headache for three to four weeks straight.

Are you then free of it for the next two weeks?

No, it may not hurt for one or two days.

So your head aches constantly?

I've tracked them. Right now, I've had this headache for a month straight.

Were you a corrections officer right out of school?

No, I worked for a bank first, a hospital television rental company, and then I decided to become a schoolteacher. I started teaching English, social studies, and math in the school for adolescent inmates in prison on Riker's Island. If they are under eighteen years old, by law they must go to school. I also taught at a few after-school programs, and summer school for a few years, then I became a corrections officer. It's a very stressful job. No two days are the same.

Have you come up with a correlation between that stress and your headaches?

When I was first hired in 1990 I was on probation for a year. It is a very stressful job mentally and physically.

You find a probation period in most jobs these days.

Yes, but this was especially stressful because I wasn't used to being around people, civilians, uniformed staff, and inmates, like the ones at Riker's. I was afraid of what might happen to me when I was inside. Unlike most prisons, we don't carry any weapons inside. Nothing. I think this is where most of my fear and stress came from as a rookie. It's just you and maybe fifty guys, or a hundred guys, or women if you're working with them. You just hope that everything is fine and that you come home at the end of the day unhurt, with all your limbs.

Does your pain interfere with your ability to carry out your job?

To an extent. Most of the time if I have a headache, I still go to work, but there are times when the pain is so unbearable I can't drive to get there. If that happens, I call in sick. However, calling in sick has many negative repercussions, so usually I just go to work and deal with the pain.

Does having the headache affect the quality of your work? Your patience with people?

Yes. It is not easy in such an environment to escape to a place where I can lie down or even sit and relax. Sometimes it just hurts to speak or hear others speak. Sometimes even the light hurts me. All those things can affect the degree of pain.

What are your responsibilities?

There are ten jails on Riker's Island, and believe it or not I've worked in all of them. We house female inmates in only one of the facilities. We also have jails in the five boroughs, including courthouses and hospital wards. All of these must be fully staffed at all times, and I can be assigned to work in any of these facilities if I am needed. My current post assignment requires me to move around a lot, escorting contractors who come onto the island, if they're going to do asbestos removal, for example. I'm also part of the Hazmat [hazardous materials] Response team, ready to respond in an emergency. I'm also trained in methane monitoring.

Have you figured out a link between your headaches and exposure to toxic substances?

I don't think so. I get tested every year, and, of course, my headaches started long before I had the job.

What do your doctors tell you is the likely source of these headaches?

Most doctors say I have migraines, but when they treat me for migraines the medications don't help. So I can't say they're migraines. As a child growing up certain smells would trigger them. If I was to go into certain department stores and smell certain odors I'd tell my parents "I can't go here, I'm going to get a headache." They used to say it was all in my mind, but of course I wasn't making them up—I really had them.

Do people at work believe your headaches are serious?

Most of the time they do. If I go into an area where people are smoking, I get a headache. If I already have a headache, it gets one-hundred percent worse. Usually they can tell if I have one because of my facial expression, or because I'm speaking very softly. Most of the time I don't tell people when I'm in pain. In fact, I have a headache right now. Of course, when I call in sick they want me to see their doctor and then they send me back to work.

Do you remember your first headache?

I don't remember my very first one, but I remember getting them quite often starting at maybe the age of five.

Do medicines help?

Some do for a few hours or maybe one or two days, but many have serious side effects. For example, the medication I'm on now causes extreme drowsiness. I don't have the kind of job where I can be sleepy. Civilians, uniformed staff members, outside agencies and so on come to the island to conduct business and work-related affairs and I'm responsible for their safety. I cannot report to work drowsy or incoherent, so I let my doctor know when I have these issues. My speech may be affected and I may experience double vision too. Anyway, this particular medication helps my headache but makes me so sick otherwise that I'm going to have to change it again.

How do your friends and family react to your headaches?

They just wish someone would come up with something to help me get rid of my constant pain. My mom is always practically in tears, worrying that I'm going to the hospital. Sometimes I just deal with it so they won't know, but, of course, the pain doesn't go away, and in the end they can see that I'm suffering. My cousin has a four-year-old. He is very aware of me being in pain. Children shouldn't have to see me like that, going into a dark room, talking slowly. My family shouldn't have to see me in pain on a daily basis. Sometimes the dark room doesn't help. Sometimes they see me wearing an ice pack on my head or my neck, but that doesn't always help either. I wear earplugs sometimes, too, when noise is a factor, but they don't always make much difference. I'm just hypersensitive to everything.

Do your doctors take your complaint seriously?

I believe they do, but they rely on various tests, and if they don't find anything on something like an MRI, they don't know what to do. One doctor said that there's marking on the back of my skull that looks like it's from an old bruise. He asked me if I was ever hit on the back of the head. My response was no, never. In the minds of some doctors, if the tests don't show anything, then there's nothing to treat. They've all just brushed me off and said I have migraine headaches.

Is it possible that you were injured when you were very small and you don't remember?

I've thought about that, and I've shown the films to other doctors, but they don't think the signs of injury are conclusive. I've also asked my parents, and their response is the same as mine—no, never!

Do you wish they would figure out something more organic, more precise?

Yes, of course. They thought it might be related to my period at one time, and put me on birth control pills. They didn't make any difference. None at all. I wish they had. Sometimes I wish they would find a tumor or something, so they could just cut it out and I would be done with it and pain free forever!

Have you ever wondered why you suffer this way when other people don't?

I've always wondered that. Always. I'm not a sickly person. The only problem I have is headaches. And they're getting worse.

When I was in high school I would have headaches, but not for a week straight. The older I get, the longer they last. But I suffer in more ways than just having head pain. I take several medications for the pain, and I can't decide to have a child while I'm taking those medications because of the danger to me and the unborn child. I would have to eliminate all pain medications to have a child and I can't imagine how I could possibly get through nine months without any medication. So thus far I've put off being a mom.

Is your pain your enemy?

An enemy, yes, but also a sign that I'm getting too worked up about things. I'm in the U.S. Army reserves, and most of the time I get a little stressed out right before my drill weekend, especially since 9/11.

What are your military duties?

My first job in the military was as a field medic. That's the same thing as an EMT. After serving for four years, I cross-trained to become a personnel-records specialist. I also currently hold the job of food-inspector specialist. To tell you the truth, now I'm thinking about getting out.

Did you have trouble getting care when you were in the army?

Yes. All they give for any kind of pain is over-the-counter drugs. They don't perform any testing. My headaches weren't viewed as anything serious, so I just did my best to handle the pain and drive on.

What do the headaches feel like?

Sometimes a pounding in the temples, on either side of my head, face or neck, sometimes a constant pain. Most commonly the pain is on the side of my head, and it feels like a big boulder is crushing it. Pressure. Sometimes it's like the pain of a toothache.

Does what you eat affect it?

Not really. One doctor told me not to eat chocolate, so I don't. Another doctor told me to try a glass of red wine with meals, but that just gave me a worse headache. I try to avoid caffeine, but it really doesn't seem to matter.

What about vacation or travel? Does the pain ease up when you're not at work?

No, it doesn't, and traveling can be a problem because my medical coverage doesn't extend worldwide. I was in Alaska and ended up in the hospital with a headache, and I had to pay for it out of my own pocket and wait to get reimbursed. Anway, they didn't know how to treat me, what to do for me. I go to Germany for my military training. When I was there in February 2002, I was in the emergency room fifteen out of twenty days. They didn't know what to give me either. Finally I just went back to work because they weren't helping me at all.

Are your headaches worse when you're tired?

I suppose my head hurts more when I'm tired. But getting rest doesn't help. I go to sleep with the headache and I wake up with the headache.

Sometimes our physical reality intrudes on our dreams. An alarm clock becomes a church bell; it rains outside and there's a storm in our dream. Do you have headaches in your dreams?

Very rarely. I don't ever sleep straight through the night, and I don't dream more than once a month. If it's more than that, I don't remember.

Can you imagine your life without this pain?

Honestly, no. I wish I could. I can't really remember what my life was like before the headaches. The older I get, the more of a part of my life the headaches become. I never thought I would get to this point where I would be in pain all the time, where I would have a headache every day of my life and that the headaches would have such intensity and duration. Really, you know what I wish? I wish and pray that someday I will be free of headache pain forever. I almost wish I could have a new head.

James Hanlon

ଜଗ

James Hanlon is an artist. For the past thirty years he has specialized in work for the Arica Institute, a group founded by the celebrated philosopher Oscar Ichazo and dedicated to personal development and world enlightenment. The images he creates have spiritual and metaphysical themes. He lives and works on the Hawaiian island of Maui. He is fifty-eight years old, and he has AIDS.

How long have you been dealing with chronic pain?
As long as I can remember.

What is your first painful memory?
My father was in the service, and I didn't see him until I was a year and a half old. I had a scar on my upper lip, and club feet. My twin sister was born cross-eyed. My father took one look at us and said, "These are not my children." That's the first thing I remember, but he beat me and criticized me throughout my childhood. I was a stranger in a child's strange land. I was isolated.

Was your father proud of your artistic abilities?
Absolutely not. I was not the son he wanted me to be, not at all, in any way. He was not in any way the father I wanted him to be either. So the source of my early pain was constant beatings. When I was nine years old I stole some money out of a piggy bank. He was in an alcoholic stupor when he found out, and he

woke me up in the middle of the night, took me into his room and beat me until my ears bled. My mother watched from her bed the whole time, screaming, but not intervening. He beat her, too, of course, but not as much as he beat me. He didn't beat my twin sister too much, but he abused her sexually. She remembers that, but she's in denial about it, so much so that when she got divorced, she went to live with him in the little town in Texas where he retired.

When did you contract AIDS?
I got it in 1984 and was diagnosed in 1986.

Are you in pain now?
The drugs I take, the AIDS cocktails, have strong side effects. I was on the first one for five years. I just started a second one. I have no appetite, I'm nauseated all the time, I have an awful chemical feeling permeating my skin and my mouth. The drugs give me terrible headaches, too.

Do you take any medications for pain?
Marijuana. It helps the nausea. It also increases my appetite, which is important because I'm just not hungry. I've lost twenty pounds in the last three months. It's very difficult for me to eat, especially in the morning, right after I've taken my drugs. I just can't deal with food. I look at breakfast and it looks like snakes to me, or insects. Marijuana helps that. I've discovered egg salad, some vegetables, soups, some fruit I like, some fish. The marijuana also takes away the pain, and it helps me mentally. It frees me from anxiety and obsession, and it frees my creativity, too. It makes me happy.

Does your art help you transcend your pain?
I've been an artist since I was seven years old, so I have to say it's been a lifelong coping mechanism for me. When I'm in my work,

it's bliss. My mind is filled with awe, with light and color and form and shape, space, time, all the elements of life. I think about the drawing, the hand stroke, the consistency of the paint, how much of it is on the brush. It takes me away to a place where there is no pain. All that exists there is my mind and my eyes. I pick up a pencil and I'm gone.

How have your caregivers treated you?

Ninety-five percent of the time I feel tremendous compassion from everyone who treats me. Once in a while, I run into a doctor or dentist who is AIDS phobic and projects his fear and anger onto me. I had that problem with a dentist recently. My father knocked my two front teeth out when I was in seventh grade, and I have to get new caps on them. Also, I have a tooth infection for which I'm taking antibiotics. I'm facing a huge bill to fix my teeth.

How do your friends deal with the nitty-gritty of your disease?

I'm lucky enough to have at least fifty really close friends. That's because of the Arica Institute, the school I've been involved with for thirty years. Everyone has been extremely supportive, more so in the old days when everyone was dying of AIDS. These days, because of the treatments, there's a bit of the boy-who-cried-wolf syndrome. Since the drugs are keeping me alive, they forget that I'm taking drugs every day and that the drugs are all that's keeping me alive. They say, "Jimmy, you look so healthy, Jimmy, you look so beautiful, Jimmy, you have the greatest constitution." They say, "we all die, Jimmy, we understand," but of course I want to wring their necks because the fact is they don't have a clue. They think they do, but they're totally deceiving themselves. Words are cheap. People can have compassion for you, but not empathy.

I worked on the AIDS ward at San Francisco General at the

height of this epidemic. I know what it's really like. You can't imagine what it's like to see someone whose body is covered with scabs, or someone sitting in a chair screaming "help me, help me!" and then proceeding to lose control of their bowels over everything. I had a beautiful lover for seventeen years who got parasites on his brain. Toxoplasmosis. He was a Yale poet who spoke five languages and translated Greek poetry. His body was totally gone, his mind was totally gone, and he wound up like a vegetable.

I've been preparing for my own death for years. I am certain that it will be a process of bliss and liberation because of all the work I've done to process my karma during my life, and all the meditations I've done. I don't want to end my life right now, or speed things up, but I'm looking forward to it when it comes. Socrates' students came to see him when he was dying. They tore their hair and wailed, and he just said, "Oh please. Give me a break. This is my liberation and my enlightenment." It will be that way for me, too.

Do you try to express that feeling in your art?

The enormous body of work I've done for Arica, which includes a tarot deck, mandalas, hundreds of dieties, has been the most beautiful and rewarding job anyone could possibly have given me. I draw spiritual characters for the well-being of humanity. The members of the school meditate on them for their own enlightenment and the enlightenment of humanity. What better job? Every day, my work is my Sistine Chapel. Even better. I'm not kidding.

You mentioned karma. Do you think of your pain in terms of karma? Do you think you are suffering because of things you have done in this or in some other life?

I don't see myself as special in any way just because I have AIDS.

We all live and we all die. It just so happens that this plague came along. We've had millions of other plagues. If it's not AIDS it's cancer. If it's not cancer it's something else. I did a meditation last weekend and concluded that Socrates is right when he says that if you've had a good life you will have a good death.

All is love, see? If it's alive, it's all God, and all God is all good; the birds, the trees, the sky. All my thoughts, all my life experience—and that includes everything I've been through—is all for the good. If that's not true, then I suffer. We have a choice. We really do. Buddha says, "all is suffering" but I don't believe that. All is love. I know that sounds airy-fairy, but it's really true. I have to look at my life that way, otherwise I really will suffer. Everything I've suffered, AIDS, my sexuality, it is all for the good because it is all about life. It's so big! I mean it's *so* big.

PART TWO

Caregivers on Pain

WHEN A PATIENT IN PAIN GOES TO THE DOCTOR, relief is at the top of his or her mind. It may not, however, be at the top of the doctor's mind. To some extent this is because many doctors believe that patients cannot be trusted to portray their own pain accurately. Doctors have been taught that pain has both a physiological and a mental component. They know that while the experience of pain can be explained by the presence of substances in the brain, the firing of specific neurons, the elaborate pathway of neural messages, and, of course, the baseline mental state of the sufferer, the experience can also be linked to the spiritual strength of the patient, his or her internal discipline, cultural background, the anchoring influences of friends and family, and last but not least, whatever emotional or financial reward—attention from loved ones, for example, or a tort settlement—the pain may bring.

The technologizing of medicine threatens to eradicate anything untestable and invisible, and because pain is, above all else, completely invisible and difficult to substantiate, it might be ignored completely if it were not so human and so devastating. Textbooks about pain written for the health care professional tend to be dry technical works that pay no more than lip service to pain's human dimension, and pain tends to be loosely appended to sickness as a sometimes irritating afterthought. Since pain has been perceived as being separate and distinct from disease, and since it is disease that doctors have been trained to diagnose and eradicate—in much the way mechanics are trained to repair a poorly-performing engine—pain has not represented the kind of solvable intellectual problem with which doctors are prepared to contend.

Ignoring pain, treating it lightly, or thinking of it only in intellectual terms defies the holistic view, transforming pain from a human experience to an academic phenomenon and thereby interfering with the trusting relationship between doctor and patient that real healing requires. While intellectual questions can and should consume the laboratory researcher in the biological sciences, the practice of medicine, some may say the *art* of medicine, must put the *patient*, not the intellectual problem, at the center of the cosmos. There are some scattered signs that this is happening. As a result of growing scientific evidence that controlling a patient's pain improves his medical outcome, the powerful Joint Commission on Accreditation of Healthcare Organizations (JCAHO), recently issued new standards for pain assessment and management, adding pain to heart rate, blood pressure, temperature and respiration as a fifth vital sign, and using a ten-point scale—where zero signifies no pain and ten is the pain of an amputation without anaesthesia—to evaluate and record the experience. Moreover, pain clinics are popping up all over the country to answer the humanitarian needs of people in genuine physical agony.

The use of strong medications, opioid analgesics in particular, remains a breeding ground for ignorance and prejudice. Many physicians, and indeed many patients and their families, are not aware of the distinction between addiction and dependence. Despite the conclusive evidence that patients in severe chronic pain do not get "high" from their medications—indeed they may complain of fuzzy thinking, constipation and other disagreeable side effects—some people still suffer needlessly rather than take medications that offer relief. Many doctors, having been scammed once or twice by a drug-seeking addict, are reluctant to prescribe such medications even when they are appropriate and required.

This situation is further complicated by the war against drugs, which makes opioid analgesics valuable street commodities, and it's made murkier still by government regulation and by new laws and legal precedents that may punish doctors for both prescribing these medications *and for not prescribing them*. With quality of life a legal issue, and drug addiction a national preoccupation, pain specialists find themselves in a nasty bind. Feeling the pressure, they want to bring their patients to the point where they can stop taking strong pain medication. Unless this is done in tandem with an elimination of the source of the pain, however, it may make things easier for the doctor, but put patients back into a state where they are unable to function normally.

The social, legal, and educational forces surrounding opioids have made it difficult for even the most well-intended physician to fulfil his professional mission, which is to relieve suffering and restore health. But while the doctor may be hampered, the real victim in all this is not the addict—addicts will find what they need on the street if they don't find it in the pharmacy—and not the doctor—the physicians lobby is among the strongest political forces in the country—but the patient. Chronic pain puts unimaginable stresses on the patient's body, his mind, and his relationship with those close to him, family and physician included.

One would hope that patients would take responsibility for their pain and seek a helpful advocate, but many lack the sophistication, self-confidence, language skills, and education to make that hope realistic. While some pain patients may be reluctant to make the point, fearing that they will be abandoned in their hour of direst need, physicians are sworn to serve their patients, not judge them. Pain control is a patient right, not a patient privilege, and treating the pain patient properly and compassionately is the healer's job. The voices in this section reflect the thoughts and actions of those on whom that duty falls.

Howard Fields, M.D., Ph.D.

∾

Dr. Howard Fields is a neurologist whose practice consists almost entirely of patients in chronic pain. At the same time, his major research interest, in his capacity as researcher at UC San Francisco, is in mechanisms of addiction. I interview him at Pac Bell Park, in between innings, as the San Francisco Giants make short work of the Montreal Expos.

Tell me how you see a doctor's role in pain management.

There are five distinct elements involved. First is the patient's need for pain relief. Second, and this is what makes it different from other types of treatment, is the involvement of the Drug Enforcement Agency, which tells you that you could potentially be put in jail if you overprescribe. Third is a law in the state (of California) that says you can be sued for malpractice if you underprescribe. Fourth there's your concern that there is no visible parameter to follow to know if your treatment is doing any good. You are completely dependent on the assumption that the patient is telling you the truth. Last, there are a few patients who will abuse the drug or divert the drug. That's a very small minority, but it does happen. So you're in a position where you have a lot of responsibility, a commitment to take care of the patient, and you must deal with multiple layers of laws and bureaucracy. It's not strictly a medical decision.

The position that a lot of physicians take is that they would prefer not to be bothered with all this, that they would rather not deal with drugs that are potentially addicting because it is a risk to them that they prefer not to have. They tend to refer those patients to other physicians who are more willing to take on that responsibility. Add to that the controversy in the field of chronic pain management, wherein there are some people who feel that giving opioid drugs can complicate treatment, and others say that the bigger problem is undertreatment and people suffering.

What is your position on that controversy?

There is really only one major problem with opioid analgesics, and that is the possibility of overdose. The way these drugs work is that they are designed to activate a receptor in your brain that normally responds to endogenous morphine–like substances called "endorphins." So what you are really doing with these drugs is mimicking the brain's normal function. If you go to very high doses of opioids, you get respiratory depression and sedation. It's very unusual. In fact, in all my years of practice I have only seen one opioid overdose in a patient who was medically managed for pain. Now, even aspirin has toxicity, in the gastrointestinal tract, and over-the-counter drugs like Ibuprofen have harmful effects on the kidneys and the gut. Opioids don't have that type of toxicity, so when I say that there really isn't a big medical downside, by and large it's because opioids are not toxic substances.

So you may ask what's the harm in using them, and the answer is that the only *medical* harm comes from this socially determined concept of addiction. In my mind, that's not something that is biologically defined, but rather means that people are taking the drug for recreational purposes. There is of course, the social harm of addiction, which consists of dropping the usual life goals of a career, family, and the broader possibilities that life has to offer—hobbies, travel, volunteer work, etc.—in favor of the all-consuming task of obtaining drugs to feed the habit.

Would you expound further on the politics and controversies of pain management?

Some states mandate adequate treatment of chronic pain, and that treatment includes the use of opiates. There's a big controversy within the field of pain management where some people say opiates create more problems than they solve and others say there's no reason not to provide an adequate dose of an opiate. And there's an additional hassle in many states, where in order to prescribe most opiates, you need to fill out a special triplicate form. The drugstores are very squirrelly about the way this form is filled out. It must be exact, and it must be presented in person. You can't telephone in this kind of prescription the way you can telephone in prescriptions for other kinds of drugs, some of which may be more toxic in the ways we just discussed. In a real sense, aspirin is a more dangerous drug than an opioid because aspirin interferes with platelet aggregation—it's an anticoagulant—and it produces gastric irritation. That combination leads to an increased propensity to gastrointestinal bleeding. If one compares the medical harm produced by aspirin to that produced by the use of opioids for legitimate analgesia, the harm for aspirin would probably be much greater.

There is a misunderstanding on the part of both patients and physicians on the risks of becoming addicted, what it actually means to be addicted, and the treatability and reversibility of addiction. Ultimately, in our culture, the idea exists that something that you just do for recreation or just do to feel good—that doesn't have any other social value—is somehow bad.

So if a patient complains that their pain isn't being controlled, they might be seen not only as a whiner, but also as someone who is indulging, by taking more opioid analgesic, in a socially worthless activity.

Some health care professionals might use that argument to justify their own reluctance to dispense these medications. It's interesting that you brought it up, because there is very much the concept of the "good patient"—the patient who doesn't complain, who just does what he or she is told and they get better. So if somebody says "Look, this isn't doing it for my pain," the tendency is to label them as weak and unworthy, and to reject them. There's also a feeling on the part of the patient of "I don't want to be a wimp, I don't want to complain, I don't want the doctor to reject me." There's that little play going on. It's part of our culture.

You say it's part of our culture. Where do you think it comes from?

Oh boy. Well, I'm a physician and a scientist, not a sociologist or an anthropologist, and what you're really asking is an anthropological question. Everybody is addicted to righteous indignation. You could say child-rearing practices are at fault. There is also this whole idea that we look up to people who sustain a lot of grief and don't complain. That's really part of our culture. The athlete who plays through pain, that's who we respect.

He's a hero even if he cripples himself.

Exactly. It's part of our mythology. And there's this demonization of opioids. I'm not exactly sure where all that came from.

Do you think that demonization has to do with the association, on the patient's part, between opioids and a terminal condition? Morphine in the battlefield, that sort of thing?

No, I suspect it's really more at the level of the great, powerful, cultural vehicles in our society: media, film, our literature, the whole idea of a counterculture as being subversive and somehow alien. It goes all the way back to [the films of] *The Man with the Golden Arm* or *Traffic*, or, if you saw it [the film], *Requiem for a Dream*. What happens is that you see the addict as a really dissolute, ruined person, someone that nobody would want to be like. There's a lot of embellishment in making the taking of these drugs somehow very lurid. I guess the purpose of that is ultimately to discourage young people from experimenting with these drugs. Obviously there's the stereotype of the addict as alien. Dissolute. In a sense, separate from society, and weird. Contrast, for example, the acceptance of drinking, in small amounts, and smoking. The media—film and television in particular—portrays these as something everyone does, as normal, as something we associate with being an adult, part of a socially acceptable icon. That doesn't extend to opiates. People who use opiates are never portrayed as part of our society.

So this acceptability extends to alcohol, cigarettes, cigars, maybe even pot, but not to opiates?

Right. Tobacco is a great example, because it's harmful. It's a toxic substance. That and alcohol are associated with large numbers of fatalities. More than opiates, at least until intravenous use became associated with AIDS. But opiate addicts go on forever. They don't kill themselves, they don't get sick as a result of the drug. Opium dens connote something Chinese, something alien. If I had to guess, the root of the demonization is something along those lines. Marijuana is not seen as a dangerous drug the way opioids are. The big argument against marijuana is that it's a gateway. That once you take marijuana, you take opiates, and that's the "hard stuff."

Is there any truth to that?

I don't know that it's not true, but I don't know of any evidence of it. If that's a gateway, alcohol is a gateway, cigarettes are a gateway. I'm just saying that part of this is socioeconomic. Who are the people who are viewed as junkies? They're not middle-class people. Middle-class people are alcoholics, or addicted to cigarettes.

Legal drugs.
Yes.

Or they're writers like me, dependent on tea.
You just enjoy the feeling of caffeine. It's not like you're trying to quit it and can't. Quitting smoking is a lot tougher, as I remember. Those are all things that go in the hopper. The other huge part of this issue is that most physicians do not know the correct dose of an opioid to use. So you'll see patients come in and say, "Oh, my doctor wrote me a prescription for a twenty-five-mg suppository, or they gave me fifty milograms by intramuscular injection. I'm still in a whole lot of pain and they don't want to give me any more." Well, what they got was a baby dose. It shows the doctor is reluctant, he is warring with himself to give it at all, but he knows that if he doesn't do something the patient, whom he figures is a complainer, will be back.

So there is a phenomenon in which a patient—who is otherwise rational and of good judgment but is in genuine distress—is in some sense set up to fall into the role of an undesirable from the standpoint of the medical profession.
This is why you're the writer. (*laughing*) You said it better than I could.

So the patient is guaranteed to fall into a nasty net if he has real pain and the physician is inadequately trained?
Exactly.

It's kind of an unfortunate dance. The doctor has one set of concerns and the patient has another.
Plus you have an exaggeration of the risk of the drug that is en-

couraged socially and by the DEA and by other people for reasons I don't understand, plus you've got some well-meaning people going around saying it's not good to give people opioids.

It's also true that there are abusers.
Yes, and they ruin it for everybody.

We need to educate patients—from octogenarian immigrants with a poor command of English to young kids—and physicians too, across specialty boundaries. A big project.
One area that this book might be able to help, particularly if some physicians would read it, is that there is this primary part of the Hippocratic Oath, which is first, don't harm. We have to redefine the concept of harm. People have to know that it is harmful to allow somebody to suffer when you have the means to end it. That is a form of inducing suffering. Really, it's mostly a sense of saying, "Look, this is your responsibility. Do this!"

Relief is what the pain patient needs. It's the doctor's job to provide it.
Exactly. It's just as important as setting that fracture. The medical profession really breaks down into two nonoverlapping camps: those who believe that the relief of suffering is their responsibility and those who think that taking care of the body is the thing, that their responsibility ends after doing physical or physiological repair.

I sense that the definition of pain is expanding.
At some level, it's very simple. They tell you, look, my pain is very bad, and you have to do what you can. You may not be able to take it all away, but you have to do what you can. That's the thing. It's just too easy for people to walk away from that, and to the extent that there are these other factors that feed into that difficulty, and people like the DEA are generating these other

factors, they are culpable. The problem is that the DEA is out of the health care loop. Nobody is making them responsible for dealing with people in pain. They can kick, and nobody kicks back.

It must be a relief for doctors to have this subject brought out into the open.
Anything that de-bureaucratizes the practice of medicine is welcome.

Othon Molina, Ph.D.

ഔ

Dr. Othon Molina is an exercise physiologist and sports medicine bodyworker with thirty years of experience. Currently, he practices on the big island of Hawaii. I interview him on Maui, where he is at work on an adventure story.

You have spent a career doing hands-on work with the human body. What perspective does that give you on the experience of pain and its treatment?

In order to talk about pain, we need to define it. There are many types of pain, many variations. Broadly, there is dull aching pain, sharp stabbing pain, cold pain, referred pain, pain from injury, pain from overuse. To treat pain properly, you have to really get to the source of the pain, and that may not be so easy. Is it a torn muscle, say, or a sprained ligament? Are your feet numb? Does this mean you have a problem with an intravertebral disc? Sometimes pain in the shoulder, in the rhomboid muscle, say, is not relieved by bodywork or physical therapy to that area because it is in fact originating in a cervical vertebra.

Each type of pain requires different treatment and assessment, which is why medications, which may be shotguns, often won't work. It's important to get a complete history, and before touching a patient, to make an intellectual assessment with questions about what they were doing just before, and at the time of, the onset of pain, even if the injury seems occult. Slowly, you narrow down the root of the pain, and then you do a physical assessment. If you think it's a soft tissue injury, you do a contraction test and then a resistance test and palpation to test range of motion.

When you take a history, what role does your take on the person's "buzz" have on your conclusion about their pain?

Some doctors believe that pain is all in the mind. My own training tells me that structure governs function. If your structure is out of alignment, your function is going to be affected. That concept applies to the mind as well as to other organs and structures.

You mean to emotions?

Sure. If the patient is in fear, if the person is angry, if the person is under heavy mental stress, the pain is going to be greater. I've seen plenty of examples of the correlation between state of mind and perceived pain.

You use massage and manipulation. Do you use medications as well?

Not at this time, although when I worked with a medical doctor, we did. I've had a chance to use both drugs and alternatives, and been able to gauge the effectiveness of drugs with an open mind. Frankly, throughout the sixties and seventies I saw drugs as the last and least desirable alternative. Now, of course, so-called alternative medicine has morphed into integrative medicine, and I'm glad to see that traditional practitioners are more open to massage, acupuncture, and other bodywork.

Did your reluctance to use medication stem from a fear that the medication might do harm, or did it stem from the belief that a certain amount of suffering was part of healing?

Quite the contrary. I feel that suffering is not part of healing. But I feel that drugs mask the true cause of the pain. I feel that doctors sometimes take a shortcut so as to fix the problem quickly, but don't take the time to assess the whole person. That has led me to my own take on pain, which is that it is a sign that something is out of balance. You can eradicate the pain, but miss the underlying cause.

Do you think that this masking gets in the way of healing as well as assessment?

Of course, because if you can't tell where the pain is coming from you can't help heal it. I've seen chronic pain patients medicated with steroids and painkillers for years so as to keep the pain at bay rather than figuring out what was really causing the pain, which was a combination of poor posture, weak muscles, and perhaps an injury that caused the body to guard itself and start a vicious cycle. More recently, though, I've seen steroids and numbing drugs actually used to do some assessment, so my mind is now open to the proper use of the proper drug.

Do you think that pain is valuable then, from a biomechanical point of view?

Sure. Pain is a wake-up call. You can have pain as light as the press of a toothpick. If you don't listen to it, it may reach the level of a ruler slapping you. If you continue to ignore it or mask it with drugs, it becomes a two-by-four wailing on you. In our society we typically wait until the two-by-four stage before we do anything about pain.

Do you suppose that's because we live so quickly that we don't have the time to properly engage and respond to our pain?

Beautiful. Absolutely. Totally right on. We move too fast, we don't have time to deal with pain. Got a headache, take a pill. Got a backache, take a different pill. It's the easy way out. I don't blame physicians for this. They are overburdened. The truth is that our educational system is weak. We are not taught how our bodies work, and we're not taught how to take proper care of them. We're not taught biomechanics, we're not taught function, we're not taught what pain signifies, nor how to interpret the message it gives us. You have to be hungry for that knowledge to find it—which often means you are in intractable pain—because it isn't easily available. Consequently, we want the quick fix.

You imply that the quick fix has a price.

The price of the quick fix is not getting to the source of the problem. Masking pain, ignoring the wake-up call, can actually cause further deterioration. If you don't listen to the first call, you'll have to listen to the next call. I've seen patients go from a manageable low-back injury treatable with massage and exercise to a severe disc problem because they didn't listen to the problem, didn't stay off their body, and covered up the symptoms with pain pills.

Of course, there are certain patients who have a very strong will. They may not be stoic, so much as determined to get better. They're easy to work with. They're great. Then you have the patients who are codependent, who have been through years of doctor visits. They are accustomed in some cases to be being pampered, to hearing "poor baby." Their favorite line is "Woe is me." They haven't really been helped correctly; they haven't really been put in touch with their own healing process. When I worked in a clinic, I lost patience quickly with individuals who didn't do the exercises I gave them. I figured that if they weren't willing to contribute to their own wellness, they weren't doing their part. Healing in a health care setting requires the practitioner and patient to work together against pain.

What would you say to the person who tells you that "Your philosophy of healing is all well and good, but I've got a job to do, children to care for," and so on?

I had that response every day, and my reply was simply to say that if you don't take two weeks off now, you may be taking ten years off later. Either heal a minor thing now, or contend with disaster later. It's very nuts and bolts.

What do you see as the social and cultural forces underpinning our attitudes toward pain, our desire to ignore it as a signal, to be rid of it as soon as possible?

The social implication of pain is quite simple, really. If you feel pain, you're weak. Nobody wants to feel that they are weak. Nobody wants to feel that they are not worthy somehow, that they are being deprived of health, even that they are being punished. Chronic pain is an unimaginably destructive experience, destructive to our sense of self. It demoralizes people. It breaks their spirit. People feel that they are less than they were when they suffer this way—less than other people, too. It can lead to suicide. I have patients who have suffered ten or fifteen years of chronic pain, and they are shadows of their former selves.

You see, ever since prehistoric times, physical survival has been of paramount importance. We had to face the tiger and beat him, and for that we had to be strong. Our competitiveness with each other comes from our deep-seated instinct to be the fittest and to survive. This is a primal drive, and pain is antithetical to it. We see pain as a failure, a weakness, an enemy we can't beat. A tiger that eats us.

So we don't want to face it. It's like sex in school in the 1960s. Nobody wanted to talk about it. Chronic pain is one of those diseases our society wants to put in the back room. We want to take it out of the social light. You don't share your pain with just anyone. It's personal. Intimate. Yet you have to embrace it to beat it.

To me, the word "embrace" connotes acceptance. But "acceptance" connotes living with it, when the real goal is living without it.

The old saw of "no pain, no gain" has caused a lot of problems in the athletic community. I don't know who invented it, but he did people a great disservice. Of course there is a certain level of discomfort that we feel when building our body, when exercising—it's called irritation and adaptability, it's the stress you put on the body to make it respond constructively. I'm talking about pain beyond this level. What I mean by "embrace" is to understand pain, get close to it, know that it's only a symptom of something else. When you have pain in the knee while running and you say, "I'm going to run through this pain," you are probably going to hurt yourself. The pain is going to get worse and worse, and you had better listen to it right away. The start of the listening process is what I mean by embracing pain. It's the opposite of denying it.

So we might substitute the word "acknowledge" for "embrace." We need to understand and respond to pain as an important signal.

If you want to conquer something, you must understand it. Ignoring it just makes it stronger. It's just like fear. If you want to beat it, you have to face it, see where it comes from, grasp it. It's a basic strategy issue. The understanding is just the first step, though. If you go to a doctor who is too busy to give you a proper work up, who just gives you a pill to make the pain go away, then you are not really ever understanding it. You're ignoring it, and you don't really conquer it that way. This takes time, of course, and knowledge.

The analogy I use is one of a car that is out of alignment. If you give it a tune-up, it will run a lot nicer. That's what acupuncture does. It tunes you up. If you go to a general practitioner you might get a pill, the equivalent of new paint or new leather—it makes you feel better but it doesn't fix that bum wheel. The only real way to fix it is to go to an alignment shop, have the thing measured, identify the problem, and true the wheel or replace it. But it's not always easy.

Yet sometimes drugs can be helpful. They can actually allow

the body to heal itself and facilitate the process. The most common structural problem in our society is low-back pain. One type is called sciatica, which may come from a disc pressing on a nerve, and it can manifest as cold or sharp or dull or numb, but the underlying cause is all the same. If I had a dollar for every patient who has ever told me "All I did was bend over to pick up the newspaper and I threw my back out," I would be a millionaire. That's how often it happens. It's a plague on our society. There are myriad events that can trigger back pain, but the fact is that anti-inflammatory painkillers, in combination with a week of bed rest, can cure 60 percent of people completely. Another twenty percent may have some lingering problem, and need physical therapy. The last 20 percent may need other intervention.

Yet a person ought to be able to bend over without hurting themselves.
Absolutely, positively true. I would love to prevent injuries that happen to athletes and other people, and we could do that through education, by teaching them proper body mechanics. Prevention is the key. But when you are a therapist in a clinic, you get the people who are injured. In that sense, all therapy is a Band-Aid. Drugs work best when you get the injury in the first day or two. If you wait a few weeks, the rate of recovery drops. The more you wait, the worse the irritation gets and the harder it is to turn it around.

The reason we injure ourselves so often, the reason we feel so much structurally based pain, is that we have gone from being an agricultural society to being an industrial society to being a technological society. We sit in chairs all day long, see? We don't exercise. We use some muscle groups too much, and others not enough. Consequently the body is out of balance.

Do you think that the principles of preparing, girding, training, and educating against injury might apply to all the different senses in which we have pain—emotional pain and spiritual pain as well as the chronic pain of disease and the acute pain of injury?

I have to say yes, I believe that. As a student of the body and a student of spiritualism, I believe that all pain comes from some kind of imbalance. Our society doesn't prepare us on all these levels though, the way some aboriginal societies did and do. We're not taught meditation, or proper communication with each other. We're not taught body mechanics; we're not taught to understand emotions; we have lost our overall balanced worldview. If we worked toward balance on all these levels, we would feel much, much less pain. If we lived the life we truly desire, we would have much less pain. Pain to me is a sign of inner struggle, our body only outpictures what is going on in our life.

Kathleen M. Foley, M.D.

❧

Dr. Kathleen Foley is a professor of neurology, neuroscience, and clinical pharmacology, and an attending neurologist at Memorial Sloan-Kettering Cancer Center. I interview Dr. Foley at her hospital office.

If a patient complains of great pain but smiles when you examine them, does that affect your sense of the validity of their complaint?

There's no question that the way a patient presents pain is a factor in how the physician assesses a patient's pain. We have a concept in our mind that patients in pain should be moaning and groaning. They should have an elevated blood pressure, and they might be sweating. We would identify that picture with pain, particularly if we could identify the source of the pain immediately. For a patient with chronic pain, the difference is that the autonomic nervous system has adapted, so the pain may not show.

So the patient who is smiling, the patient who is able to sit in your office for thirty or forty minutes without moving in the chair and describe to you the burning sensations that she has, the hyperesthesia that she has, the changes in sensation, the severity of the pain, that patient makes you then sit there and say, "How should I believe that she is in pain?" That's a construct that most clinicians go through, and we have to sit back and remember that this is subjective phenomenon, and that it is what they say it is.

The difficulty that we come to is what to do when after a full

113

evaluation, the patient has a normal exam, has normal X rays, and yet complains of symptoms. Is she in pain? The reason I'm emphasizing this is that working in a cancer center, you often come across people who have early disease that you can't find on their exams and you can't see on their X rays, and yet they complain of pain. Then, three or four months later—and I've had a lot of experience with this—their bone scan or their MRI scan evolves to really show something. It's so humbling to realize that I may not have believed them, I may not have listened to them, I may have judged what they were saying. That kind of experience makes you extraordinarily humble when people tell you about their pain, because it may be way beyond what you know, and way beyond what anyone at that time can know.

It also becomes very obvious that when we have a patient with a pain complaint but no objective radiologic finding, even if he has an abnormal exam, we spend a great deal of time talking about the patient's psychosocial issues. But when we have a patient with a tumor invading his bone, we don't talk much about his psychological state, because we can immediately correlate his pain to that site. The dimensions of our ability to assess pain are complicated by the fact that this is a subjective experience, and that we professionals tend to objectify it, and when we can't, we minimize it. This is a serious problem for the patient with pain.

Especially when they know that people respond with greater credulity to someone who is wincing and huffing and puffing than someone who seems dispassionate and cool in describing their own symptoms. That must put the patient in a balancing act not so dissimilar from the doctor's, in which the patient wants not to appear to be making too much of something, but at the same time wants to communicate, using cues that any outside person would respond to, that they are hurting.

I'm not sure about that. The public at large is much more generous about pain than medical professionals, because they don't have to treat it. They don't have to contend with the complaint and do something about it. I must say that I'm quite amazed by how tolerant people are when someone says they're in pain. Nobody questions it in any way, shape, or form. They believe it. So the greater burden to the patient is that we professionals have to make judgments. The family member or the friend has only to be the family member or friend. In those roles they can be the patient's advocate, but they're not put in a position of having to judge anything. Rarely do family members come in and say, "We don't think he's in any pain." They definitely come in and say, "We don't think he's telling us about all the pain he's in. We think he's trying to protect us from that. We think he's struggling. We think he's trying to fight it." Often they say, "If I were in as much pain as he is, I couldn't possibly do that."

Pain is one complaint that everyone else is so afraid of. Especially if they've had any experience with it, they're extraordinarily respectful. So pain is the one thing that the public will give a person the benefit of the doubt about, because it taps into their own extraordinary fear of pain. With that comes a sense that they shouldn't underestimate or undertreat pain in someone else because that someone else could easily be them.

One might not think that the health care professional—motivated in their career choice by compassion and an interest in helping others—would be tougher to convince than the public at large.

To be a competent physician means to identify a cause for the pain, to relate the symptoms with something concrete. If you look at the history of medicine, clearly we made a major shift in how we dealt with symptoms for patients when we professionalized medicine. Initially, medicine was no more or less than the treatment of symptoms using opioids and a whole variety of other agents whose mechanism of action was unknown. We had the application of a wide pharmacopoeia of nonspecific and specific treatments for symptoms.

Then, in the latter part of the nineteenth century, when physicians were thought to be quacks and medicine strongly needed to professionalize itself, the American Medical Association fostered the Pure Food and Drug Act, to advance the science of drug therapy. The number of Americans taking analgesic drugs, particularly opioids, was high in the late nineteenth and early twentieth centuries with the professionalization of medicine and the organization of the pharmaceutical industry. Drug therapy became focused on disease, not symptoms. In the last twenty years we have begun to refocus on certain symptoms, like pain, and refocus on the scientific basis of pain. When it comes to treating patients in pain, particularly with opioids, we are thwarted by our lack of knowledge of the mechanisms of pain relief. There is a lot of mythology and not a lot of clinical science, and politics are coloring things at the present time.

We know that for the cancer patient we have had a natural experience of using opioid drugs clinically. This clinical experience has demonstrated the safety and efficacy of opioid drug therapy on a chronic basis. Yet we don't have good studies. We have a lot of indirect information. At the same time, this is not taking place in a vacuum, but in a society where the misuse of prescription drugs and the abuse of illegal drugs are our American disease. We are in this culture of drug abuse that has little to do with the patient with pain and everything to do with opioid drugs and everything to do with a fear of drugs and with a lack of science and an unwillingness to support the clinical and research effort needed to change our knowledge base. The question is, why is that? What is the problem? What would keep any doctor from adequately treating a patient with pain? How powerful must these forces be? Much as we have identified what the social barriers are, we haven't identified the personal barriers of physicians.

It strikes me that the physician's job is not to sort through all the political and social issues surrounding drugs, but rather to remember the oath they took and treat patients in the most compassionate possible way. My bet is that if the other issues were released to public forums—voters and referenda and such—the result would be better medicine.

You probably could argue that point. I get a little bit worried about compassion. There might be many physicians who are compassionate but wouldn't have a clue about the right drug to give a patient, and the right dose. Thinking it was the right thing to do, they might give too little or too much. Compassion is not a bad thing, but I would want to temper it with knowledge. You could have the most compassionate surgeon but he could do the wrong operation. Compassion isn't the first word that you would want to assign to a physician. I would want to assign competency first. What we are struggling with now in our society, in our technological revolution, is how do we expand the role of that physician to include issues of empathy. This is well recognized as the whole conceptualization of humanism in medicine. How do we now bring that back in as part of our technological revolution? With all of these drug treatments that we have, with all of these approaches for patients, the goal of the physician as a compassionate ally to patients is less important. We have a drug that can make them better tomorrow, so we don't need someone there holding their hand.

But if you have nothing to do for a patient, if you have no treatment, then it is important. This has been so well described recently in the AIDS epidemic. If you read the autobiographies of physicians who worked from the first days when there were no treatments to now—when we have extraordinary treatments to prolong survival—you see this transition from the physician who spent a lot of time talking with the family in a psychosocially empathetic fashion to a physician who hands the patient his regimen and doesn't talk to the patient. So I would argue that we may soon become extraordinarily good at treating pain, and that may have nothing to do with our compassion, but everything to do with our extraordinary competence. If I have a patient with trigeminal neuralgia, and I give them an antiseizure drug that dramatically relieves his pain, compassion doesn't need to play a role.

I guess I see a larger role for compassion.

I worry about compassion; it can trivialize the scientific basis of medicine.

I can't help but think that medicine exists only to serve compassion. The notion that compassion could trivialize medicine startles me. I'm more worried that medicine will trivialize compassion.

I wouldn't even begin to argue that compassion is what moves people to achieve competence. But should compassion be what makes a cardiac surgeon know how to do an angioplasty? Of course not.

Clearly you need both.

You need both. I worry about too much competency without compassion, and I worry about compassion without competency. They need to be balanced. I don't think that my plea to the deans of medical schools about pain management should be on the basis of compassion, but on the basis of competency. There is a science; there is a knowledge base; there is a very serious public health problem; and pain management should be taught in medical school. Will it make physicians more compassionate? Ideally.

Would it make them more sensitized? Ideally. But we didn't set up medical schools for compassion.

There we have the kernel of the issue.

That's why I worry about using the term "compassion" in the pain arena, because it makes it just that you're doing good without a more detailed expansion of what that means. For doctors, they're not just doctors to do good, to be good; they are doctors to have certain skills, to have a certain level of professionalism. I'm really pushing this. It's a battle I fight a lot.

It's an interesting and key battle. My sense of this is that one should not be a physician in order to have a skill set and be competent. My sense is that one should be a physician to do good. Skills and competence are just tools that allow the physician to do so.

Absolutely. But in the pain arena, where we are dealing with subjective phenomena, we minimize the importance of the science of pain, the knowledge base we have, by saying, "Just be a compassionate physician and everyone will be better." That's garbage.

If I have neuropathic pain as a result of having injured my leg in an accident, I come to you, not my shoemaker, because I expect that you will have competencies that my shoemaker does not, but I still expect you to be highly motivated to help.

There are times when I don't have any way to help, and this example you picked could be one of them. At the moment, as it happens, we don't have good treatments for neuropathic pain. That doesn't mean that I can't compassionately say, "This is a terrible problem. I wish I could make it better for you; I wish I could take care of you for the rest of your life, but I don't know how to help you. But there are some things going on, some studies, some trials, and there are some things we can try."

What you've described sounds exactly like a partnership of compassion and competence. We can't always find a magic wand to make things better.

Right. You can't always make it better, but you can acknowledge their pain and suffering, and care for them.

The patient who comes to someone like you, a specialist in an august institution, surely does not want to hear that you can't make them better, because they don't have anywhere else to go.

The most honest statement may be that you don't have a silver bullet, but you do have things to try, and that you'll take care of them. One of the greatest difficulties we see with patients with pain is that physicians might not feel responsible for them, might not see value in a therapeutic relationship with a patient that is based on doing nothing, or on a therapy with opioids, and might therefore say, "I have nothing I can do for you, so good-bye."

Wendy Lazar, L.M.T, C.Ht.

☙

Wendy Lazar is a certified hypnotherapist, and a massage therapist working in Boca Raton, Florida. She has had a number of careers and business ventures before becoming a licensed therapist— including a stint as a private investigator—but describes herself as a mind/body integration therapist. I interview her over lunch.

Give me an example of how hypnotherapy might help somebody in pain.
I had a lady who was referred to me for regression therapy through hypnosis by a medical doctor in Miami. The doctor called me and said, "Listen, I hate to present it to you like this, but I have a nut on my hands. I don't know what kind of voodoo you do, but you help these people." The patient had undergone gallbladder surgery, and had been suffering intense postsurgical pain for over eight months. She had seen many doctors, but nobody could diagnose the cause of her pain, which had started when she left the hospital.

Did someone leave a sponge inside her?
That was exactly what she was concerned with. She had all the bloodwork, diagnostics, scans, and therapy ranging from orthopedic workups to chiropractic, and nobody could find a thing wrong. When she came to me, she was crying. She said, "I tried to get exploratory surgery, but my surgeon wouldn't do it. I know he left something in me. I know there's something going on. What do I do?" I questioned the surgeon, who reported that

121

everything had gone normally. I asked him if he played music during the procedure, and he said no. I asked him if he talked about golf, or about anything else in particular, and he said there had been nothing unusual, that the whole thing was no big deal. I told the doctor: "Allow me to remind you of the power of the spoken word." Actually, I had warned him of this before.

So I regressed the patient. Now the way this works is that I help the client relax as much as they want to, and ask them to be in touch with the emotion related to their situation. I follow along and ask them what's happening. This woman took me back to the operating room, and she became hysterical. She was very fearful. She didn't want to deal with it. So I emerged her from the regression. We talked about the tremendous fear she felt, and she told me that her father had had what was supposed to be a simple surgery and he had died. We talked about that for a while, and then I sent her home.

A week or so later, she came back and told me that although she still had the pain, she felt hugely emotionally relieved. We went back to the surgery again, and this time she allowed herself to experience it. I asked her who was there, how many physicians, and I asked her what they were saying. We went through almost two hours of things that were being said. Finally I told her to move to the point where they were about to remove her gallbladder and asked her to tell me what was happening then. She told me that one surgeon was making fun of the size and condition of her gallbladder, and then she told me that the other surgeon exclaimed, "Oh my God, she'll never be the same."

I asked her how she felt about that comment, and she said it was going to ruin her for life. I asked her how pain played a part. She said, "Well being ruined has to be painful." I asked her, "Who says it has to be painful?" She said, "It's surgery." I said, "Who says surgery has to be painful?" She said, "Well, my father died." I said, "Oh, okay. I get it." Then we worked on forgiveness and setting free, trying to comprehend what the doctor meant, exploring the possibility that he might have been trying to say that once he removed this organ that was causing her so many problems, she would be much better.

I'm amazed that she was able to hear what was being said during surgery.

You can hear when you are under the effects of anesthesia. You are not deaf. Your conscious mind is asleep, but your subconscious mind can hear and record everything. So when she emerged from her regression, she said, "I think that's it. I trusted him so much that I was convinced I would never be the same." I told her to rest, keep a journal, call me in a week or so and tell me how she was feeling. When she did call back, she told me that she no longer had pain. I said "Wonderful! Anything else come up?" She said "Yes, I've been having vivid dreams of my father. I haven't dreamed of him in years."

At that point I sent her to a psychologist. They worked on the emotional aspects surrounding losing her dad so suddenly, and distrusting the medical community. I did some additional work with her as well, saying good-bye to the gallbladder, bidding it farewell, and filling that area of her body where she felt there was now a void. She didn't know what to fill it with, and I asked her if self-love might be an option. That helped enormously. She went back to the surgeon, and she gave me permission to tell him what she had learned. I talked to him too. He thought we were both crazy, which is okay. He and his colleagues had prescribed pain medications and antidepressants for her without result, and I felt that was the wrong way to go.

How do doctors find you?

Word of mouth. I'm known as the witch doctor who can handle

the crazy people, and I figure that's fine. I'm willing to try to help patients even after physicians have given up on them.

If physicians think you're a witch doctor, I'm curious to know what you think of their pain management practices.
Some doctors think their patients are histrionic and ignore pain complaints. Others think their patients are manipulative drug seekers, and others are just legal drug pushers.

Give me an example of a legal drug pusher.
There was one physician who referred to me for quite a while. A patient would come in complaining of pain, muscle spasm, insomnia, or depression and without blood work or diagnostics, she would prescribe narcotics after a five minute interview.

Our health care system does not encourage lengthy history-takings and extensive consultations. What do you suppose might be a doctor's motivation for behaving the way you've described?
I'm sure that much of the time it's about making money as quickly as possible, but in all fairness, this physician I'm speaking of had her own pain, and it was emotional.

So it was uncomfortable for her to deal with the pain patient?
Very uncomfortable. Her entire mantra was "I just want my patients out of pain." I think what she was really saying was "I just want to be out of pain myself." So her intentions were probably good, but in my opinion, it wasn't the best way to deal with it. It wasn't the *medical* way to deal with it.

Does your regression therapy include regression to past lives?
I regress people to the cause of what brought them to me. Usually there are serious emotions involved in regressing to the cause, and we go back to the very first time they experience those. I don't lead them, I follow them. It's a journey through the per-

manent memory of the subconscious mind, which I've been taught to believe is our self-preservation mind. All the information is there. What the conscious mind of the individual will allow them to recall may be another story, because the conscious mind protects by analzying and rationalizing the discoveries a person may uncover and what they can handle in one sitting. If they are truly ready, and their conscious mind realizes it, they expose it. If not, it is saved for another time.

So if they believe that their headaches come from when they were Cleopatra and an asp bit them on the nose, you don't care, so long as it helps them be free of it?

It doesn't matter to me where they go or what they tell me about the cause. It's not for me to judge their experience. One specific case does come to mind. It turned out to be an apparent regression to a past life. There was a woman who was having neck pain, and she did not have a great range of motion in her cervical vertebrae. Her family was wealthy, so they were able to pay for many different types of therapy over many years. By the time she got to me, she was fifty-two. I regressed her to the cause of her pain, and she took me back to when she was a child in this lifetime. I asked her whether it was the first time she had felt this particular pain. She said no. I asked her to go back to the original time, to the initial sensitizing event.

What made you think that what she described was not the original event?

The fact that when I asked her whether it was the first time she had felt the pain she said no.

So what was the first time?

When I asked her to go back to that, she started speaking another language. Now this was a Roman Catholic woman who was very devout in her religion and was very apprehensive about hypnosis to begin with because of the implications.

You mean the notion of past lives and reincarnation?

Subconsciously, perhaps. So when she started speaking this language that was unknown to me, I didn't know what to do. I had never had that happen before. I asked her to either call in an interpreter or interpret herself, so that I could understand what was being said.

What language was it?

Latin, but not the modern form. She went back to another time, when she was a man. She was being hanged for having an affair with a woman who was married.

The reason for the sore neck.

Absolutely. She had a great deal of guilt as she was hanging there. She, or he, knew what he had done and felt remorse. I asked her what this had to do with the person who was sitting in my chair today and she said, "I have to forgive myself." I said, "All right, are you willing to do that?" She said yes. I asked her whether there was anything else we needed to do? She said, "I have to make amends with the gentleman whose wife I had an affair with." So we asked him to come in, and she spoke with him, and there was forgiveness and she was set free from both the physical and emotional aspects of her pain. Then she told me she had to come through a tunnel with light in it, and be born to the mother and father of this life. After the regression I sent her to a physical therapist who worked on her neck, and in about seven or eight weeks she had complete range of motion and no more pain.

Any other examples come to mind?

Yes. One time a man came to me for pain in the right jaw. I moved my hands over his energy field for problems as I prepared to treat him, and I felt that something was amiss in his left ankle. I asked him whether he had a problem there, and he told me that he had recently had surgery on the ankle to repair a fracture. I asked him when he had started having the pain and he replied that it was shortly after he was in the hospital for surgery on his ankle. I felt there was a link between the two, so I suggested we regress him. When we did, he recounted his operating room experience. Again, I say that while the conscious mind may be asleep, the subconscious hears and records everything. While the patient was sedated, the surgeon took a look at his ankle and said, "What a nasty break. The line of it reminds me of this jaw fracture I heard about last week."

What led you down the road of helping people in this way?

I know I am here to be part of the solution, to help assist others in their healing. I've wanted to do this kind of work for as long as I can remember. I've always wanted to be the helper. I am the youngest child of a family with four children. My mother and father never divorced, but probably should have. Dad was an alcoholic/rage-aholic and mom was, for lack of a better term, codependent. When I was twenty-seven, my brother was murdered. He was a drug dealer, which is why he was killed, but he had been to a regression therapist and had kicked his habit after just three sessions. Thank God he died straight.

I thought my life was over when that happened, but as it turned out, it was just beginning. I couldn't help anyone then, not even myself. I went through a lot of spiritual revelations and emotional growth, from wanting to give up on life and leave the planet to knowing that I could not, that I had to stand up and face the music. I tried regression, too, and learned that my initial sensitizing event had to do with my father. It was in another lifetime, and I was my father's mother. In order to rise above the anger and disappointment that I felt for my father I suppose I had to go to this other time where I was rocking him as my infant son. Experiencing that, and coming through it back to this time—whether it was a true past life or an ancestral memory didn't matter—took my pain away. That was when I began to study mind/body therapy, learning to integrate regression with hands-on therapy, which is what I offer people who come to me for their pain.

Modern medicine makes a distinction between physical and mental pain. What insight has your professional experience given you regarding that separation?

In every individual I've worked with, and in myself, the mind/body link is complete. Every regression that I've ever done has always gone to an emotion. We truly are psychosomatic beings, in the sense of linked mind and body. We all have painful things to work through.

David Seidenwurm, M.D.

༚ড়

Dr. David Seidenwurm is a Stanford and Harvard University–trained neuroradiologist working in Sacramento, California, where he specializes in MRI and CAT scans, spine injections, and other tests. He is an editor of the Journal of Radiology, is on the editorial board of the journal Diagnostic Imaging, and was until recently on the clinical faculty at University of California, San Francisco. I conduct the interview at his home, while his two young daughters play in the other room.

Can you see pain on a film?

Absolutely not. A film can look perfectly normal and a patient can have excruciating pain, or a film can look completely abnormal—someone can have a spine you wouldn't wish on your dog—and they can be completely fine. The thing that always surprises me as a neuroradiologist is what is normal. What's abnormal, that never surprises me anymore.

How do you define normal?

Normal is a funny word, isn't it? Confusing, too. Most people think that normal means perfect, but I'm forty-four years old and I've got crow's-feet and gray hair and that's normal for me, but it wouldn't be for a twenty-year-old. We work with three meanings of normal in medicine. First is normal distribution, as in the average person, the "picture" that you would see in the average forty-year-old person, the average fifty-year-old person. Normal also means perfectly free of any defect. Another meaning for normal might be a patient with no symptoms.

Let's explore how this relates to the pain patient. If you read a film for another physician, and that physician tells you that his patient is in great pain but you don't see anything on the film, what conclusion are you likely to draw?

I'm likely to think that there is something that I'm not seeing, and that the technique that I'm using is fallible. The patient who is in pain is always going to get attention. If someone has taken his complaint seriously enough to send him for an MRI, someone is going to take good care of him. Frankly, what I'm much more concerned about are the people who have minimal symptoms, and who, because of some legal agenda or just to cover the bases, are actually made ill by findings on a scan that deviate in some minor way from perfection but may be demographically normal for their age group. That's a much, much, bigger problem. Let me give you a scenario. Someone overexerts himself, strains his back lifting something at work, or is in a minor fender bending car accident. He might feel a bit stiff for a day or two, or even for a week or two, but there hasn't been any important damage to his spine. Through the workman's compensation system or the legal system, however, he is sent for a scan and that scan shows findings that a normal middle-aged person could have, a narrowing of a disc space, for example, or intervertebral disc degeneration. A disc bulge. Even a small disc protrusion.

So someone might have a minor work injury, and he has an examination, a lot of Latin words are used, a 3-million-dollar machine shows some abnormalities in his back, and presto, he has a structural totem and becomes focused on his pain. An MRI can help to restore walking to the lame in some cases, and it can take a perfectly healthy person and have her driving down the aisle of the grocery store in one of those electric tricycles. People become fixated on the findings, because it is produced by a technological marvel. They don't trust the doctor, who understands the variability in populations and has the training and experience to distinguish a minor injury from a serious one.

All this suggests that you believe there is a great deal of correlation between the mind and body in the experience of pain.

There's no question about that. Yet society teaches us to ignore those connections, and no one is taught that more than the neuroradiologist because we focus on the structural causes of pain. But really, it's important to understand that just because we see something that might be a deviation from perfection, that doesn't mean that it's a cause of pain, especially when normal subjects with no pain, scanned as part of research studies, exhibit those very same findings quite frequently.

What do you figure is the unknown factor that determines whether or not there is pain?

One factor is the mind. We know we can be distracted from pain, that easily verifiable structural injuries hurt less when a person's attention is somewhere else. We know that pain hurts us more at certain times of the day and maybe not at all at other times. Stories of someone not noticing a bone sticking out of their leg when they are in extremis, in an accident say, or preoccupied with the welfare of a loved one, are quite common. The experience of pain can be affected by what other people say, too. If someone tells you that you have what looks like a terrible injury, it's likely to hurt more. If someone says that your injury looks like nothing, you're more likely to just get on with things.

We are never amazed by a picture that shows an abnormality causing pain. That we can understand. But the two things that perplex us are when we see a normal scan in a patient with pain, because it shows the inadequacy of our tools, and of course we are surprised when we see abnormal scans in study subjects who have no pain at all. So let's say we take a picture of a tumor of the larynx for cancer staging and we obtain an image of the cervical spine and we see bones protruding into the spinal canal, or we see the spinal canal narrowing, and these patients have a hoarse voice and a lump in their neck, but no pain. Or let's say we are studying a patient for gastrointestinal symptoms and we do a CAT scan of her pelvis and her abdomen and see her spine and there are disc herniations or severe spinal stenosis and yet she is completely asymptomatic.

How do you explain that?

As part of the variability of the human condition. The cancer, for example, may have grown in a period of months, but bone changes take much longer, which tells us that the bone changes must have been there before the cancer and yet there was no complaint. So for pain to occur, you need the perception of pain, you need the pain to play a role in your life, and you need, presumably, some anatomical or biochemical substrate for that pain.

What sort of role might pain play in life?

The most crass of course might be when someone is in litigation and being in pain is going to make him money. He may hurt because he got a lot of attention by hurting, and the lawyers would be disappointed if he stopped hurting—the system seems to have an interest in keeping them talking about how much they hurt. Also, pain can make a person feel dependent, and some people want to feel that way. Certainly the medical system itself fosters dependence on itself.

Sometimes patients are frustrated by negative tests when they're in agony, because they are looking for their pain to be validated. What should a patient make of a negative test?

It could be that it is the wrong test. It could be that it is an inadequately sensitive test. But assuming that the doctor has done his job properly and the machine has functioned properly, patients should be happy that they don't need an operation to take care of their pain and that some other approach to their pain would be more beneficial. They should be delighted that there is nothing compressing their nerves, that there is no tumor in the canal. They should be glad they can be treated conservatively.

It always strikes me as odd when someone's test is normal and he's disappointed. You're giving him good news: They have no mechanically crippling condition, no cancer, whatever, and yet they seem unhappy about it. I understand the validation question, but I've never really gotten a handle on this.

Maybe a variety of approaches have been tried to heal the patient or at least make him comfortable, and those approaches have failed, and the patient is hoping for some diagnosis because even a scary diagnosis is better than none at all.

Unfortunately, it's very difficult to achieve total mechanical clarity all the time. It's ironic.

Do you have thoughts about the intricate dance that goes on between people and their doctor in terms of discovering the source of their pain?

Sometimes our goal as doctors is not so much to discover the source of pain as it is to find a list of things that are *not* causing the pain. I used to get pictures sent to my laptop computer at home over the teleradiology network. My daughter was about five years old at the time, and I would sit her on my lap and show her the images and teach her what to look for. Then I would call the hospital and she would have to say, "No mass, no bleed." Eventually she got to the point where she would look at the scans all on her own and put her hand on her hip and say, "No mass, no bleed, huh, Daddy?"

One time they sent me a scan of the abdomen. My daughter looked at the scan and said, "Daddy, that's not a brain. What do you want me to tell them there's not?" So a lot of radiology is telling other doctors what there is not, so they can go ahead with less mechanistic approaches to a patient's pain rather than one that is based on a tumor or a hemmorhage or some other condition that requires emergency surgery.

Have you ever had a scan for your own pain?
Yes. I had some back pain four or five years ago.

How did you contend with it?
Activities of daily living, and an over-the-counter pain medication. It turns out that for low-back pain, the activities of daily living are as effective in many people as physical therapy. The Finnish garbagemen study shows that. Some Finnish group randomized Helsinki garbagemen with back pain into three groups; one got bed rest, one got physical therapy, and the last group was given time off work but was told to just go live their lives. It turned out that the physical therapy group and the activities of the daily living group did better than the bed rest group, but those two groups did about the same.

Did you find yourself hoping for one result or another from your own MRI?
Oh, I definitely wanted normal. Are you kidding?

Gerald Young, M.D.

꙳

Dr. Gerald Young runs a pain practice in Soda Springs, a rural town in Idaho's Southeastern Bear Valley. His facility abuts the local hospital. On the Internet, he refers to himself as the "Chief of Troubled Waters." I interview him in his consulting room.

Is running a pain clinic a lucrative proposition?

The answer is that it depends upon the kind of practice you choose to have. For people who do procedures, it probably is much more lucrative than a regular medical practice. Doctors in the trenches—primary care physicians, internists, family docs—don't do as well. If you have no conscience, you can see an enormous number of people in a day in a pain clinic. It can be an assembly line, with people lined up around the block waiting their turn to get a prescription for pain meds. Naturally, such a doctor can give pain medicine a bad name.

Personally, I find it impossible to practice medicine this way. Morally, ethically, and legally it's wrong, and more important, this type of practitioner violates a basic precept of medicine by not having the best interest of the patient anywhere in sight. I try to take a lot of time with pain patients. Those who see my practice as an enormous waste of time, who don't see the value in taking care of pain patients, simply don't understand the problem. These patients have an incredible number of needs in addition to obtaining a prescription for pain medicine. They need to be told that they're okay as people. They don't just come to my clinic to get pills. It goes a lot deeper than that. I'm sure you've heard it said a thousand times—show me someone in chronic pain and I'll show you someone that's depressed. Chronic pain patients have had every bit of dignity and self-respect they've ever had sucked out of them by the system. For some folks it's easy to lose sight of the fact that with rare exception, not a single one of these patients began their life in chronic pain. They had productive lives at one point; they took care of their own problems and the problems of their family before the monkey of chronic pain climbed on board. Then their life unravelled, and pain and depression crept in.

Would you talk a bit more about the link between pain and depression?
There are two kinds of depression. The chemical kind, where neurotransmitters have gone awry and society has beat you down and the stress of it all has taken all you have to give. That kind of depression responds very well to antidepressant medications. Then there's situational depression. It's not so easily treatable. Until the situation changes, the depression won't change. For many chronic pain sufferers, the situation is not going to change. The medicines cost a lot of money. It costs a lot to see a doctor. Most of these people can't work any longer. They don't know where the money's going to come from. These folks live a depressing life. There isn't any long-term hope for them. Sound depressing? It is.

Some people are lucky enough to be able to afford to go to the pain clinic up at the University of Utah. I see them when they come back, and they're higher than a kite on themselves. They feel so good about themselves, about their pain and all the ways to deal with it, but they've just had occupational therapy and physical therapy and psychological counseling and all these people to buoy them up. The resources at the University of Utah's pain clinic are endless. The patients return home looking forward to trying different approaches to pain, to avoiding the drugs, and then they get home and they're alone in rural Idaho without any support system at all. After about two weeks, reality hits them in the face and they realize that life ain't so grand. All they're left with is the fact that medication relieves the pain. So they try to get on some medication. If they have to make a financial choice among types of medications, they'll choose the pain medicine, because it gives them the most relief. So it turns out this isn't easy. It's damn hard. It's a depressing, depressing situation.

It doesn't sound like the system helps as much as it should.

People in chronic pain are suffering through a chemical situation where nature's morphine, the endorphins, are depleted by what they've been through. They generally run into a continual stone wall in the system. The doctors expect them to jump through numbered hoops—this test and that test, this consult and that consult—before they can get their pain medicine. Then they have to go to the pharmacy, where, with rare exception, the pharmacists fall in step with the medical practitioners and make the patients feel like dirt under their feet. So by the time these people get to my office, they have been reduced to the lowest level our society has. For, you see, they are now identified as being addicts.

Let me tell you a little bit about the pharmacy experience for pain patients. I have a friend who has severe chronic low-back and leg pain as a result of degenerative disc disease, spinal stenosis, and three failed back surgeries. One day he had me go to the pharmacy with him. He had told me stories about the treatment there, but I didn't believe him. Anyway, we went, and the pharmacist glanced at the prescription without making eye contact with my friend or acknowledging his presence beyond putting the prescription on the back counter and muttering it would be a while. After forty-five minutes or so, he called my friend back up and handed the prescription back and said, "We don't deal in this kind of medicine. We don't treat addicts. You gotta try the methadone clinic. If you need this garbage, try getting it off the street—that's where they sell dope."

It was the most incredible experience I've ever had. This patient looked like anything but the stereotypic image of an addict, if there is such a thing. He was polite, the prescription was written by a licensed physician in an appropriate dosage, but it was the kind of medicine that the pharmacist immediately associated with addicts and abusers. The pharmacist treated him in a way that people simply should not treat other people.

What do you think makes people treat others this way? What do you suppose it is about an opioid medicine that brings out this bias?

To answer that, you have to look at the roots of our profession. In medical school, attitudes in pharmacology are opinionated and derisive toward this kind of medication. They carry on through to internship, residency, and out into practice. And at the same time, they are reinforced in nursing school and pharmacy school. As you may have guessed, in terms of the way they treat people, the toughest ones out there are the pharmacists. But the more I think about it, the more it strikes me that it starts even before one's professional education. It is ingrained in us from day one that people who take opioids are bad people. I remember the movie *The Man with the Golden Arm* with Frank Sinatra. People think that's the kind of abuse we're talking about here, and it isn't.

When you think about it, this whole "just say no to drugs" thing is also about saying no to medication. We're raised with the attitude from the time we're old enough to watch TV. It's a cultural thing. Street drugs, drug use, addicts, those things have a powerful negative connotation. And the government is part of the problem. Government spends a lot of money trying to stop illegal drugs and money coming in, but that's too hard, so they pick on the doctors and the pharmacists. We live in a computerized world. It's easy to count prescriptions, and when federal agents need trophies for the drug war, doctors are easy pickings.

This whole negative attitude toward pain medication changes, of course, the moment severe chronic pain touches someone. Then, in the twinkling of an eye, they are able to open their mind about the benefits of opioids and see the legitimate side of it. That's the only side of drugs I deal in. The legitimate side. But it's so hard to legitimize the subject. People almost have to experience it to understand. The understanding comes when someone's life is ruined by chronic pain and the right medication helps him or her put it back together. Then the light goes on and the thinking of opioids as being something bad is reversed and the "good side" of pain pills can be appreciated.

Do you have any examples to share of patients who were poorly treated before they came to you? People who were allowed to suffer needlessly?

I had one just this morning. A fellow in his mid-sixties came in suffering from polymyalgia. He's a retired gentleman who has gone from riding his horse and helping friends work their cattle to not being able to get out of a chair without excruciating pain. He is waiting to see a specialist, but he couldn't get an appointment for two months. His therapeutic medicine didn't work, and he didn't have anything to take for his pain. What was he supposed to do, just suffer for two months until the specialist could see him? I couldn't allow that. I'm sure I'll get castigated. I'm sure the specialist will tell him I'm everything but a legitimate practicing physician, but I had to give the guy pain relief. Hell, if what you're doing isn't helping and if you can resolve the thing, why should the patient have to suffer? That's one thing I haven't figured out. *Why* should people have to suffer until he can arrange a consultation with a specialist? The prevailing attitude in Pocatello, which is my referral center, is that you have to learn to live with pain—it's part of life. My question is why? Why, when we have medicines that can control it?

You need to understand that my first move when I see a patient is not to reach for narcotics. Before a patient is admitted to chronic pain management with opioids, he undergoes a thorough workup of his problem. I don't hesitate to refer patients with undiagnosed illness that involves pain. The point is to try and find the organic cause and cure that and the pain with it. Opioids are used only when there is nothing further that can be done to relieve nonmalignant pain. This is a point I make over and over again. Why should a patient be abandoned at this point? No further tests to do? Fine. No further therapeutic options? All right. Then give the patient a life with pain relief. If it requires opioids, then use them in the dose necessary to control the pain. Just don't abandon these patients!

You can have people sign medication agreements—we don't call 'em contracts, but that's what they are—you can have them go only to a pharmacy of their choosing, and you can control exactly how much they're getting. You can do drug screens to see if they're taking anything else. Currently, I don't have one single patient in my pain practice that I'm worried about taking anything else. These are just average, everyday people who have been dealt a dirty blow by life, had an accident or something has gone wrong and all of a sudden they can't provide for their family, they can't go to work, they feel they are worthless, society tells them they're worthless, and they have chronic pain on top of it. By

God, I can't turn my back on people like that when I know there is medicine that will make them feel better!

It seems awfully simple. People are suffering, and you undertook the job of helping them out. Somehow that fact seems to have gotten lost.

The only thing simple about what I just said is me. I'm trying to present this complex issue in a straightforward manner. Right now I am lucky enough not to have any patients that I'm worried will take some other drug, but physicians have to be constantly on their guard for abusers, and also not be too quick to label patients as drug seekers. By the time patients come here for pain relief, most of them have been to specialists, had all kinds of tests, and so on. To some extent they know how the game works. They know the answers they have to give in order to get the pain medicine. Some of them have become deceitful. Some of them lie to you. All most of them are trying to do is get relief. They've been forced to act dishonestly by the system. They're used to it. People perceive them as being drug seekers. They're not seeking drugs, they're seeking relief from pain. They're pain-relief seekers. That's all those pain pills mean to them. They are pseudo-addicts. They exhibit drug-seeking behavior just as a true addict does, but they're seeking pain relief, not a high.

Opioids can be dangerous drugs, but they have legitimate uses, and they are nothing short of miraculous for those who need them. Usually for the treatment of chronic pain you give them a long-acting opioid, and then a rescue medication, a short-acting medication, for the bad days or the bad times. Interestingly, I almost never see anyone come in to get a refill on their long-acting medication that doesn't also need a refill on their short-acting medication—their rescue medication. Nobody ever seems to have any rescue medication left over at the end of the month. Perhaps what happens is that since these people are never free from pain but have the pain made tolerable by the long-acting narcotics prescribed, if they see some leftover rescue medication as the month winds down they figure, "Why not"? Let's see if I can be pain free for a day or two or an hour or two. Then they come in with the empty bottle. It's always an empty bottle.

Shouldn't they be given what they need to be pain free all the time? I mean if you drove your pickup truck into the service station with an empty tank and told the guy to fill it up and he said he'd only give you six gallons, you'd ask if there were a shortage. If he said no, you'd ask if he was worried you couldn't pay, or that you'd drive off. If he said no again, but still insisted on only giving you six gallons, you'd drive out of there in a huff and find another station. You'd never accept such poor service in a gas station, nor in a restaurant or a department store, but in a doctor's office, where you or your insurance company are paying for a much more important service, you are forced to smile and say thank-you to this kind of treatment. Seems outrageous, and yet we accept it. Why do you suppose that is?

You just entered the world of the chronic pain patient. That's what every one of them looks at; having their medicine titrated down. Doctors ask, "Don't you think you could cut back on this? Don't you think maybe you could cut the dose down?" What they should be asking is, "What is it going to take for you to be as pain free as it takes for you to be functional?"

The spectre of the DEA might hang over doctors on this one. They're willing to jump into the game, but only up to their ankles or knees. Instead of jumping in all the way and getting the job done, they do a little bit and figure it's better than nothing. Very few doctors look to titrate up to where the patient says, "Hey, this is great! I feel good!" If the patient says they feel good, it's time to titrate down! That is medicine as the chronic pain patient sees it. My God, they're almost afraid to say they feel good because the first thing the doctor is going to want to do is cut their medicine. It's appalling to see how these people are treated. It's disgraceful! They never get to the level that they really need, and if they do, their doctor cuts 'em back. If they need so much it makes 'em sleepy, well for God's sake there are things that can keep them awake, too. Say that to the average doctor, and Great God Almighty, it's heresy. They'd castrate you for it.

Why can doctors get away with it but a gas station can't?
Supply and demand. It's hard to find a pain doctor, a prescriber. The doctor may have an idea ahead of time of what he's going to give a patient, and if the patient doesn't like it, isn't grateful, the doctor can just tell them, "If you don't like it, go someplace else!" So the patient has to say "Oh, thank-you, Doctor! I appreciate you, Doctor! You're a marvelous physician, Doctor." And then as the patient is out the door, he's calling you a miserable son of a bitch, and he's still suffering. The fact is, it's doctors' egos that are the problem. They have to be the ones making the decisions. If the patient suggests adjusting the dose, the doctor feels he is losing control. Doctors are not programmed that way. The pain patient's feedback, his desires, his wish to be free from pain, can't enter into the bargain.

You've said that doctors who write pain medications are called "prescribers" and made it sound as if that's a bad word. Do doctors have pejorative terms for patients in pain?
A "prescriber" is a physician like me. I am not strictly a pain doctor. I'm not a pain specialist. I am just a family doctor who has practiced for a long time and one day finally saw things for what they were. I decided that if I could help chronic pain patients and do it in a legitimate way, with help from consulting specialists where needed, and if writing Schedule II prescriptions for patients who need them were the area I could make my contribu-

tion, then that's what I would do. No, it's not the same thing as finding a cure for cancer, and I doubt very much if doing this gets me much respect from my colleagues—in fact I take a lot of criticism—but that's okay because I'm doing the right thing.

As regards undiagnosed patients who suffer chronic pain, yes, doctors may label them unkindly. If a complete history is performed and a thorough physical examination is performed and if the appropriate tests don't reveal the etiology for the patient's complaint, then obviously there's nothing wrong. It's in the patient's head. Doctors call those people "crocks." Unfortunately, in chronic pain, scans and so on don't always show what's going on. So it's left to the physician, and you either believe them or you don't believe them. Some prescribers may write meds a little too easily, and some doctors don't write them easily enough. For some doctors, it's a badge they wear. They won't prescribe Schedule II substances. They're hot shit. There are neurosurgeons who won't even write for postoperative pain medicines. They leave it to the family doctor. They won't dirty their hands. It's the biggest bunch of bullshit I've ever seen. It's okay with these guys if the patients get the medicines, but they're not going to be the prescribers. They act as if this makes them better, but it's two-faced. It's hypocritical. I have a hard time with doctors like that.

You have clear opinions about some doctors.

When you come out of medical school, you feel like you're a child of a higher god. You're taught to feel that way, and your patients reinforce the feeling. They tell you how great you are. Pretty quick, if you don't watch yourself, you begin to believe it, too. You see yourself as a special person. You think you're a little bit higher up on the food chain—that you don't make mistakes. At this point the doctor is just about to commit the biggest error of his career in medicine—he is about to stop listening to his patients and begin relying solely on himself. Lord deliver me from that kind of a doctor. We're not so great. We're just people. But some doctors can't see that.

Maybe the whole problem of the inadequate pain management boils down to the intersection between cultural prejudice and medical education.

It does. And the victim, as in all things in medicine, is always the patient. Not the drug companies, not the DEA, not the doctors, nurses, or pharmacists, but the patient. If anything goes wrong, it's always the patient who pays the price. And he pays the price big time in the pain game—perhaps the most tragic patient experience in American medicine today.

James S. Hicks, M.D.

ೞಖ

James Hicks is an associate professor of Anesthesiology at Oregon Health and Science University in Portland, Oregon. We meet at his office in the hospital.

Tell me a bit about your background.

I trained in obstetric anesthesiology at the Naval Hospital—San Diego, then did a tour of duty in Puerto Rico. After the Navy I went to a county hospital in the San Francisco Bay Area, working in a Stanford-affiliated teaching position. After that, my wife and I spent eighteen years in the little Oregon town of La-Grande. I joined the army reserve there, went to Desert Storm, and eventually got command of the reserve hospital in Vancouver, Washington. I became interested in medical administration while dealing with the Oregon Health Plan, and got a master's of medical management degree from Tulane. I moved to Portland a few years ago, and before I had this job, I took on the medical directorship of the Board of Medical Examiners, the arm of the state that licenses and disciplines physicians.

What sorts of issues did you deal with in that latter capacity?

Prescribing problems associated with prescribing for chronic pain, for one thing. I learned about the intractable pain law, a safe harbor for physicians who took care of chronic pain patients who did not have cancer, allowing them to prescribe without getting into trouble. This was important because a few years earlier some

146

important people were saying that there was no place for opioid therapy in the management of chronic pain that was not due from cancer. During my tenure, the BME was transitioning from a position of disciplining prescribers of long-term opioids to accepting the position that indeed there *is* a place for properly managed long-term opioid therapy there.

In what way are you involved in this area now?

As a paid lecturer working for a pharmaceutical company, I go around the state talking to physicians about what the BME expects. It's not rocket science. It's third-year medical student stuff. You take a history, you do a physical examination, you make a diagnosis, and then you make a plan. That plan may entail surgery and it may involve opioids, but it is not one in which the patient comes in, says she has pain, gets a prescription, gets another one two weeks later and so on until finally you quit recording any physical findings on the patient and just refill. The board won't tolerate that. It's not the management of pain. I urge doctors to go back and think about the way they were taught to treat diabetes, to diagnose its often insidious onset, to examine the systems it affects—the circulatory system, the neurological system, the renal system. You formulate a plan that involves insulin therapy, diet, and so on. I urge doctors to take that same reasoning and apply it to chronic pain patients. You don't just refill insulin over and over.

You've made an interesting analogy between pain and diabetes. It suggests that you see pain as a disease.

Physicians will diagnose failed-back syndrome as something you treat. Failed-back syndrome is not a diagnosis. There is a tendency to confuse symptom and diagnosis. It is important to establish a true diagnosis. Chronic pain is not a diagnosis. It's not in the patient's best interest to be sequestered under that rubric. These patients have specific management needs. Frequently they have lots of psychological overlay or multiple diagnoses, including depression. That depression may be primary in the sense that it allows the pain or associated condition to become worse, or secondary, the result of the pain itself. In a comprehensive pain center, it is important to have people who are skilled in isolating the various components of pain, including body mechanics and mind mechanics, psychology and physical therapy, and the actual somatic lesion that must be considered. Consider all these things in concert and you're doing it right.

So the nub is establishing a diagnosis?

Exactly. You take a history, you do a physical, you establish provisional and differential diagnoses, and then you start a treatment plan. That plan may require more diagnosis, surgery, physical therapy, and so on. Then you go back and assess how the patient is doing. You don't just say, "Here's your prescription." You try to get to the root cause. If those causes are not fully treatable and you still have residual pain after treating them, then you treat the pain itself. You don't just treat pain for pain's sake. You have to know what's producing the pain to the greatest extent you can. Sometimes all you can do is narrow it down and do a trial of opioids, keeping good records. But the key is to see the patient regularly, to establish a diagnosis. The State of Oregon also requires you to do two other things. You must get informed consent, and you must get a consultation with an expert in the part of the body that is considered the source of the pain. You want to recognize that chronic opioid therapy has risks, and therefore, before you commence it, you want to make sure that the risk/benefit ratio is the best it can be, and that it is clear to the patient. You want to rule out less expensive, less invasive, less risky treatment modalities first.

Too, when you do use opioid analgesics, you want to use the right ones, in the right manner, on the right schedule, and teach the patient pain management, not just throw them a prescription. You have to teach a pain patient how to manage pain just the way you teach a diabetic how to manage his blood sugar. A typical, well-managed pain patient on opioids will be on a baseline opioid and a rescue drug, which can be used to manage extra stresses, like exertion. There's a band in which they know they can function, but this needs to be taught. It's not instinctive.

At this juncture it might be good to remind ourselves of the distinction between addiction and physiological dependence. Very few people actually become addicted. One definition of addiction is the use of antisocial, unaccepted, or illegal methods of obtaining drugs. A lot of patients on opioid therapy are physically dependent on that therapy, which is to say that if it is withdrawn, there will be symptoms, and those symptoms will be more than just the return of the pain. There's nothing wrong with dependence. Those of us who drink coffee are physiologically dependent on it. If I haven't had my coffee by ten in the morning, I'm looking hard for it. The truth is, I might even do something mildly antisocial to get it. We all have our little dependencies. But street addicts, those who rape, pillage, and plunder in order to get medications, are the rare case. They are also the people who have never had chronic pain. Most addicts are not chronic pain patients, but many well-managed chronic pain patients may well be physiologically dependent. Many people use the word "addicted" too loosely, but even physiological dependence was considered unacceptable in the past. Over the last several years, dependence has become more accepted, particularly when the patient has been educated in pain management.

Is it the responsibility of the patient or the physician to manage pain properly?

It's a shared responsibility. One of the two state requirements, as you may remember, is informed consent. The notion of that in Oregon is that you advise the patient of the risks of opioid therapy in the same way that you would advise him or her of the risks and benefits of having a gallbladder removed as opposed to treating it medically, or of having a cosmetic procedure as opposed to living with wrinkled eyes. You must make clear the material risks associated with the use of opioids, including side effects such as constipation, blurred vision, dizziness, perhaps the inability to operate machinery or drive, although many people can drive on these therapies. When there is true pain, the proper amount of opioids will attack the pain before they attack mentation.

So the responsibility is shared, but it depends upon teaching?

Many physicians execute an opioid contract with their patients, an express agreement where a patient agrees to see only that doctor, to get prescriptions only from that doctor. The patient will not spill thirty tablets down the commode, give it to the dog, augment it at the emergency room, and so on. If the patient violates this agreement, the physician will no longer care for him, no longer prescribe for him.

The carrot and the stick.

The carrot and the stick.

Steven Graff-Radford, D.D.S.

ଔ

Dr. Steven Graff-Radford is a dentist by training. He runs a head-and neck-pain clinic at Cedars-Sinai Hospital in Los Angeles. I interview him over a Japanese lunch.

Would you begin by sharing your vision of pain?

It's too simplistic to say that pain is just a process of electrons that travel along the neural system or nociceptor. It's a multidimensional problem, and it evokes a change in human function that most people have never witnessed and never can understand. Part of the reason our society has ignored pain is that in reality it's a symptom, and is therefore considered a nonserious process. It's considered something that doesn't kill. It's considered a process we are left to our own devices to deal with. It's partly based on the loneliness that's created in society. We isolate ourselves, and we're taught that we really mustn't reveal too much to the people that we're around because of the competitiveness of society. Therefore we don't reveal our pain, whether it's physical or emotional, and we don't investigate that pain.

When pain patients describe their symptoms to me—for example, a throbbing headache or a pounding headache with nausea and light disturbance, and I say, "How is your relationship with your mother?" they may burst into tears and answer, "You know, you're the only doctor who's ever listened to me." Well, maybe I'm not the only doctor who has ever listened to them, but maybe I just asked the right question that day. Sometimes patients react differently. Sometimes they say, "Look, you're way off, this is just purely physical, so why don't you just give me a magic bullet?" They don't want to deal with what the emotional aspects really are.

Where were you trained?

At UCLA. I was the third dentist ever trained in this country in pain management. But pain management has blossomed over the last twenty years in this country. I used to go to American Pain Society meetings and find only two or three hundred people at a meeting. Now, thousands go to these meetings. There has been a huge, dramatic proliferation of literature and science and processing the understanding of nociception, but in reality it speaks to our lack of empathy that so many people are ignored who have chronic benign pain and that sort of process.

Is it really true that symptoms are not able to kill? What about a heart attack?

You don't die from the pain. You die from the fact that the heart has stopped functioning. The pain was just the signaling system that took you to the doctor.

But there appear to be people who are in such intolerable pain that they kill themselves to be free of it.

I think it's premature to go as far as euthanasia for pain. Far, far, far too premature.

I wasn't advocating any such thing. I was just trying to draw a connection between people seeking to end their lives and the intolerability of their pain.

I think I agree with that. Patients with pain are unbelievably desperate. They are underestimated: not taken seriously. And there is something very interesting that is evolving. A majority of patients in pain clinics are female and suffer from fibromyalgia, migraine, chronic fatigue syndrome. In the past there were other fad-type diagnoses—Epstein-Barr virus, those sorts of things.

When you say "fad" do you mean they don't exist?
Just that they didn't sustain themselves. Probably because we didn't understand the symptomatology and that became the label for those people who were suffering at that particular point in time. With science, we prove that they don't have a virus, but we don't prove what they do have. There's some new literature on what's called "stress analgesia." When you stress an animal, it becomes analgesic. So you take a rat and make it swim in cold water and it becomes analgesic. It's like having a motor vehicle accident. You become analgesic. You don't feel the pain of the accident, so that you can cope with it.

You go into shock.
You don't want to call it that, because "shock" has a specific medical definition. But this analgesia is reversible with noloxone. Do you understand the concept? This is an opiate-mediated analgesia. So what I'm saying is that you take an animal and you stress it. It becomes analgesic, and you can reverse that analgesia by giving it noloxone. That suggests that it's an opiate-mediated analgesia. The noloxone reverses the effect that the stress creates.

Why would an opiate reverse the effect?
Because what's happening is that the body is actually creating endorphins that bind to the receptor and the noloxone knocks out those endorphins. Now if you take the same animal and put it in warm water for three minutes, it becomes equi-analgesic, but the effect is not noloxone reversible.

There's another mechanism at work.
Right; reversible this time by a drug called MK801, which is an

MMDA antagonist. The point is that you have opiate and non-opiate mediated analgesia caused by stress, by swimming. This is not true with female rats, because in the face of estrogen, female pain inhibition is inhibited.

There are a bunch of new studies showing that if you injure a nerve you get a higher incidence of what looks like neuropathic pain, nerve-generated pain, in the presence of estrogen. If you take male animals and female animals and you injure them equally, the females have more hyperalgesia and neuropathic-type symptoms. You take out their ovaries and it drops down to the same level as males.

Would this be adaptive for, say, childbirth?
Good question! In childbirth, estrogen levels drop down to almost nothing, and you have normal analgesia. When you start to think of concepts like this, you see how little we know about the overall function of the brain. We tend to write things off and say that women are complainers, or that women do this or women do that. So if you exclude behavioral factors, you ultimately make a mistake.

So are we heading toward a model of pain management that is multi-variate and multidimensional?
We should be, but we're not. As a society, we are doing exactly what I started off saying we were doing, which is that if we can't find a neuron or electrode to switch off, then it's your fault, pal, so deal with it. Once again we isolate the pain patient more and more, and the more you isolate the human being, the less he or she can function, the more he or she suffers, and, ultimately, kills him- or herself. My ultimate goal would be to consistently remind people that our goal is to understand the nociception. You cannot divorce yourself from the fact that the emotion is very important.

Whose goal? The researcher's goal? The doctor's goal?
The doctor must understand the nociception to treat the pain.

But he must also understand the other variables.
Exactly. And equally! Equally, if not more.

You mentioned the competitive nature of society. Could one contend that it is adaptive in a Darwinian sense to be able to deal with pain better?
I would assume that pain is on the uprise, whether it's emotional or physical, based on the fact that our goals are not really to take care of each other, but to defeat each other.

Isn't it time for the artificial distinction between mental and physical pain to go out the window and a new, tertiary model be evoked?
Absolutely. In fact the definition of the term "pain" needs to go out the window, too. The International Headache Society and the International Association for the Study of Pain define pain as an emotional experience expressed. They use that word. Expressed. So what if you're deaf, dumb, blind, whatever? Can you not have pain?

If you can't express something, that doesn't mean it doesn't exist.
Right. If you're an animal and you can't express it in human language, does that mean you don't have pain?

I suspect that the population at large, people who have been in pain or have had loved ones in pain, do not perceive the medical establishment as having an enlightened view.
They don't, and I don't think the medical establishment has an enlightened view at all. Most pain physicians are nociceptive physicians, because ultimately, how do you make money? You write drugs or you do procedures. To sit down and talk to people for hours not only doesn't make you a lot of money, but it takes a whole lot of time, and half the time you're going to piss off your

patient anyway! They didn't come prepared for that, expecting that. They don't want me talking to them about that, even though they and society need something more cortical, more emotional.

I read a lovely book that described a young kid, a student, who had won a scholarship and was pre-med at Stanford. He did so well, that, in his third year, his father gave him a gift for getting straight As and sent him on a trip to China or wherever, and over there he met a guru who told him, "You're wasting your time. You shouldn't be so caught up with competition. Everything in your life has been this competitive process. You should join the ashram." So the kid writes that he's not returning home and about eight months later writes again. "Everything's so wonderful," he says. "I don't compete anymore. I'm having such a great time. I'm closer to myself and I feel wonderful and real and everything. And by the way, I'm currently second in my class, but by July I'm sure I'll be first!"

I often say that when I'm old and gray and able to retire, whatever that allows you to do, I would like to answer one question. Or try. I've often discussed this with a rabbi. Why does it take pain for society to learn?

I would counter with the question: Why is it that individuals appear to learn from pain, but society doesn't?

That question is a very good starting point for someone who wants to be in pain management. It shows the complexity, the hugeness of the problem. That's why I think so many people die in pain. There are so many unanswered questions that people have in their lives.

Grace Forde, M.D.

Dr. Grace Forde practices at the Cohn Pain Management Center in Bethpage, New York. The center is a part of the North Shore–Long Island Jewish Health System. I interview her at her office.

Tell me a bit about your practice.

We draw from all of Long Island, Queens, Manhattan, Brooklyn. I even have patients in Florida and one patient in Israel. This is an interdisciplinary pain center. A lot of places call themselves that, but we really are. We do physical therapy, biofeedback, massage therapy, interventions that include triggerpoint, botulinum toxin and epidural injections, psychotherapy, even acupuncture. The number-one diagnosis we see is lower back pain. That's a multifactorial condition that usually involves degenerative disc disease and sometimes a secondary myofascial component. Number-two is headache.

Botulinum toxin sounds like what causes botulism.

Botox. Yes. It prevents the release of acetylcholine. That's the substance muscles use to talk to each other. The toxin helps them relax. It decreases the spasm, which can be very painful but is usually secondary to whatever else is going on.

You used the term "intervention."

These are mostly injections and other basic procedures for the relief of acute pain, but also spinal cord stimulators and opioid pumps for chronic pain.

How did you get into this field?

That's an interesting question. I'm a neurologist. I did my residency at the University of California, San Diego. Patients with chronic low-back pain were always sent to the neurology clinic, but no one wanted to see those patients. I thought that was totally unacceptable, so I started to see the patients, and after a time they were sent to me by default. I was a resident in neurology though, not pain management, and I didn't feel that I knew what I was doing. So I did a one-month pain fellowship elective at UC, San Diego, and learned aspects of anesthesia. I did it for a second month, and I decided it was what I wanted to do. That's how I got into it. Nobody else wanted to treat these people.

Your description of your education suggests that there was the discipline of neurology and the discipline of anesthesiology, but no separate discipline for pain. Is that changing?

Yes, but ever so slowly. In medical school you rotate through other specialities, but not, in general, through pain management.

Why did people at San Diego turn their backs on pain patients?

Because they are difficult and demanding patients who complain all the time. They hurt, and they want you to know it. They make your life miserable. But you have to understand that they are difficult to manage because they are hurting. They're anxious and they make *you* anxious.

Helping people who are hurting is why one becomes a doctor, no?

You would think so. But chronic pain patients are very angry. They're angry with the world. They feel, "Why me?" They can be very verbally abusive. On occasion these patients come in and meet me for the first time and start yelling and screaming right away. I have to tell them, "Wait a minute. I know you're angry. You've been treated badly in the past, but I'm not the one to blame. We have to start afresh." You calm them and then you can get through to them. There's a lot of frustration at having been ten different places and not having been helped.

Why have they been treated so badly in the past?
They've been treated badly because their physicians don't know what to do. I can't speak for all physicians, but a lot of physicians feel impotent when they don't know what to do to help and then they blame the patient. They think "It's your fault. I'm a healer and I'm supposed to heal. If I can't heal you, something must be wrong with *you*—not with me." That's what we're taught in medical school, and if you have that mentality, then pain management is not the specialty for you. In this field, you rarely heal folks.

You're taught to expect cures in medical school?
Not in the curriculum exactly, but you pick it up from other physicians. You have appendicitis, you go in, the doctor takes out the appendix, you're cured. That's the sort of thing physicians like. There's a beginning, there's an intervention, there's a resolution. In chronic pain, that doesn't exist. Most of these patients say things like "Stress exacerbates my pain." Some physicians may think, "What a crock." Or the patient may say, "If it's going to rain the pain gets worse," and the physician may think "Gee, maybe he's crazy."

But it's acknowledged that stress does exacerbate pain, and barometric pressure changes may, too.
Absolutely. But that is something that we are just now coming to believe. A lot of physicians didn't believe that before. Same thing with menstrual migraines. Some women experience worse headaches around the time of their period. Unfortunately, and I'm not trying to be sexist, a lot of male physicians still do not

believe, even in this day and age, that there is such an entity as menstrual migraine.

You mentioned that you do acupuncture here at the clinic.

Yes, I'm a licensed acupuncturist. Most patients are not satisfied with only Western treatment. Quite a few came to me and suggested I do acupuncture. They said their insurance company wouldn't pay for it unless an M.D. performed it. Enough patients suggested it, so I did it.

So it was a patient-generated ambition.

It really was. I went to Los Angeles and did a four-day course, then did home study for six months, a *lot* of videotapes—forty of them, each two hours long—then I went to Atlanta and did ten days of intensive acupuncture, and then I was certified at the end of that period.

Do you use it often?

Not that often, because it is very time-consuming. You can see from that stack of charts there on the table that I have thirty-five patients scheduled for Monday and to do acupuncture you need to put in the needles and let the patient "cook" for maybe half an hour. I don't do a whole lot of it because of time constraints. I do research and see patients. I just don't have the time.

Is acupuncture effective?

You have to choose the patients carefully, as with every other treatment. It doesn't work for everyone, but for some folks it works. Lower back pain may respond, as may headaches and musculoskeletal pain. Some people go on and on and on, but I do eight to ten treatments. After those, if the patient hasn't gotten any better, I stop. For migraine, I do mostly physical therapy and botox. Botox is very effective.

When chronic pain patients come to you frustrated and angry, do you think of them as whiners?

No, I do not. If you take the time to find out, you discover that not all chronic pain patients, but a fair number of them, have childhood traumas such as physical, sexual, mental, or verbal abuse. This is especially true of patients with gynecologic pain, chronic abdominal pain, and disorders like that.

So psychological issues manifest physically as chronic pain?

In some people, yes.

Are there more female chronic pain patients than male?

More patients are women because women tend to seek medical care more than men do. It is often the woman who drags her husband to the physician. I think women are a little bit smarter than men in that sense. (*laughing*) We complain a lot, we cry a lot, and maybe that's why we live a little bit longer.

So men are taught to keep a stiff upper lip?

Absolutely.

Is it harder to get a man to admit he is in discomfort?

No. Interestingly enough, by the time they come to me the patients have already admitted that to themselves. This is a tertiary center. It's a last stop. There's no pretense here. A woman will sit here for an entire interview and cry. A man would not do that. But I have a way with patients, and I get them to tell me everything that's going on, much more than I really want to know a lot of the time. But that information is important. Patients don't live in a vacuum. Everything has an impact on their pain. I want to know about their home life, their job, everything that's going on. Patients open up. They spill their guts. If these walls could talk, you would be amazed at what they'd say.

So pain is a multidimensional phenomenon.

Of course. It affects every aspect of a human being.

When you say that pain affects a patient's whole life, I can't help but wonder if it isn't also true that every aspect of their life affects their pain. Isn't it a two-way street?

It is. Lack of sleep, for example, increases the pain. Anxiety increases the pain. Sometimes patients use their pain to do something or not to do something. Maybe a husband only pays attention to his wife when she says, "Gee, I have a headache." Sometimes we see that.

What about social isolation? Isn't it also true that people don't want to be around patients in pain?

Naturally, they don't. People in pain aren't nice. They're angry. Sometimes a husband will come in specifically with his wife to tell me how difficult she is to live with. He'll say, "Excuse me, but she's a b____ when she's in pain." So then I have to explain to him how the pain affects her mentally. He came to hear that there is really something wrong with her and for her pain to be validated to him.

And depression?

Depression is part of the picture. We've had two patients who committed suicide. One woman put a gun to her mouth and blew her brains out; the other took pills. Very traumatic.

You felt you had done your best to help them and there just wasn't anything to do?

In the case of the one who took the pills, I felt that I had done my best, but after she passed away her mother called and said, "She really liked you, but you guys missed the boat. She was very depressed for weeks before and nobody picked it up." The patient was on antidepressants, and I thought she was getting better, but what the mother said was really hard for me to take, because I thought I was doing everything. It hit home very, very hard.

And the other suicide?

I didn't have a clue. She was young and she had chronic pancreatitis and was on a pain patch. I saw her about a month before. She said she was doing fine, said her pain was better. The next thing I heard, she blew her brains out.

I've heard that's a very painful condition.

Just like the acute pain, except it doesn't pass. It goes on and on with no end in sight. It wears you down. It decreases your ability to cope until you just can't deal with it anymore.

Opioids wouldn't help?

The patch was delivering opioids. Just not enough. Not enough. Very sad.

What I have noticed with some women with chronic pain is that they have very low self-esteem. I'm not quite sure whether the pain came first and the low self-esteem followed it, or the other way around. I've seen some of these women stay in abusive relationships because they think that somehow they deserve the pain—that they are supposed to suffer for some reason.

A lot of people write on their patient questionnaires that their religion, their faith, has sustained them, but I can't really say I believe it. It may be lip service. The way people react to pain is definitely a cultural thing. I'm certain of that. I am from Trinidad originally, and I've noticed that a lot of people from the West Indies don't want to complain. We are supposed to be strong. We are supposed to take whatever comes our way, suck it up and move on. We don't want to be seen as weak, so we just move on. I know that because I do that myself.

So you take a patient's cultural background into account when evaluating their complaint.

Absolutely. I saw a woman from some South American country, I don't remember which one. She'd had migraines for thirty years. She had a thirteen-year-old daughter, and she didn't want her child to see her suffering, lying in a dark room with a pillow over her head. She came in here and felt safe enough to cry. She cried her little heart out right here in the office. I needed a truckload of Kleenex. Afterward she looked at me and said, "That was the first time I've let go. I can't do that at home. They don't understand."

I've heard a lot about the importance of validation. It seems that it is almost as important as physical relief.

It absolutely is. A lot of people come in here and say "Thank God someone finally believes me! I'm not alone with this anymore." It's amazing, but a diagnosis has the power to make them feel better. That and spending time with them, holding their hand. I do a lot of hand-holding over the phone. When I give a patient their medication I tell them to call me anytime, twenty-four hours a day, seven days a week, if they have problems. I find we can talk on the phone and it's helpful, especially when I'm trying to get them off medications that may even be causing their symptoms, especially migraines. To tell you the truth, a lot of times they don't even call, but just knowing that they can goes a long way.

It sounds as if validation is a medication of its own.

It is definitely therapeutic sometimes.

That doesn't say much for our culture—that we should live in such a way that nobody has anyone to talk to, that people are suspicious of each other, don't believe each other.

No, it doesn't. I give lectures all the time. Last night I was in Detroit, and my opening line was "You have to believe the patient."

You see, pain is always, always subjective. If you start out with the premise that someone is trying to hoodwink you, you should refer them to someone else. You are not the person to treat them. A lot of times physicians worry that patients are just drugseeking, that they are just here to get medication to get high. If you start from that premise, the game is already lost. You need to refer that patient on. I start all my pain-management lectures by making this point. You have to believe that the patient is suffering, even if his pain is mainly psychological. Psychological pain can manifest physically. It happens a lot of times.

Of course, the distinction between psychological and physical pain is one we concocted. It doesn't exist from an experiential point of view, and pain is a word that describes an experience.

Physicians often tell patients that their pain is all in their head. Well, of course it's all in the head. You have to have a brain in order to feel pain. So it is all in the head. That's where pain is felt.

But that doesn't make it any less real.

Not at all.

N. Gregory Hamilton, M.D.

⚷

Dr. Gregory Hamilton is a practicing psychiatrist and the cofounder and past president of the Oregon-based Physicians for Compassionate Care, an organization that alerts the public to the dangers of the assisted-suicide movement and educates health care professionals in treating patients nearing the end of their lives. He is also the author of several books on psychotherapy. I interview him at his office in Portland, Oregon.

Are people who want to die, like those assisted by Dr. Kevorkian, victims of inadequate pain management?

Dr. Kevorkian is in jail, and that is where he needs to be. What he was doing was evil. He murdered people. The pain-control movement was coopted by radical, suicide-on-demand proponents who espoused the notion that people should be able to kill themselves whenever they like, and should be helped to do so. Here in Oregon, we have made good headway raising the level of pain medication we use—as measured by the DEA statistics on per capita morphine use. Our numbers continue to go up. Unfortunately, the assisted-suicide movement has portrayed the end-of-life as being a choice between going gently or dying in some kind of inescapable trap of grotesque, burning agony. That movement did nothing to help pain care and pain management.

Are you saying nobody was moved to suicide by intractable pain?

There have been no cases of people seeking assisted suicide being primarily motivated by intractable pain here in Oregon. They've been motivated by other factors: fear of loss of autonomy—not by loss of function, but fear of loss of function—fear of being dependent on their families, fear of being a burden to their families, and, of course, they've been motivated by depression. There are documented cases of people who were given assisted suicide instead of treatment for their depression.

Now, there have been a few cases of people who listed, way down on the list, the concern that they might, in the future, suffer untreatable pain. But basically, we can treat pain. We have had national expert after national expert come out to conferences here in Oregon and talk to the doctors, nurses and hospice workers about pain control. These experts basically say that pain is treatable, and that people do not need to die in unrelieved agony. Depression is treatable, and opioid analgesics, surgical and radiation procedures, anti-inflammatory and antispasmodic medicines are all very effective in pain control. When we systematically treat people's fear and pain both, people do not have to be frightened into assisted suicide.

What does the term "pain" evoke for you?

That's a complex question. Pain has to be assessed in the same way as any other problem in medicine—biologically, psychologically, socially, and spiritually. Each of those dimensions can be addressed in a way that helps people dramatically. We've already talked about medical options. Psychologically, pain is augmented by fear, abandonment, loneliness, feelings of disconnection. People need to have a sense of control over their pain. They need to feel understood and cared about. Socially, people need company, and they need someone to suffer vicariously with them, to empathize, to not only relieve the pain, but to say, "Whatever happens, I'll be here with you." They need others to witness their suffering. Spiritually, people need help understanding how they can find meaning in life despite the fact that life includes loss and suffering. A religious community or spiritual practice makes people much less likely to despair, or think that they can't tolerate pain, and that hedonistic comfort is the only good thing life has to offer. There are multiple causes of pain and its perception, and there are multiple remedies.

Would you address the physician's role as witness to suffering?

Everyone wants a compassionate physician, and the fact is that most physicians are compassionate just as most people are compassionate. We may hide our feelings behind a professional demeanor or scientific thought process, but no matter how cool we seem, we see our patients and we suffer empathically with them. That's what "compassion" means. With passion. Suffering with. Physicians want to help. The medicines and techniques we have available make that possible, and the physician's caring helps the patient, too. We can't make people live in a pleasurable state all the time. There's a limit. We don't really want people to be high all the time anyway, and people generally don't want that themselves anyway. But they don't want intractable suffering either. They want to be able to function. They want to live their lives. There have been very good studies to show that empathy, witnessing, reduces the amount of pain medication patients need.

It sounds as if you're saying that when the patient feels good, the doctor feels good. Yet physicians often don't prescribe enough pain medication. Why is that?

Physicians are as compassionate as anyone, but like everyone, they have their shortcomings. As a group, physicians have great difficulty with feelings of helplessness and lack of control. When physicians come to me as patients, those are the major issues I have to help them with. A minority of outliers of the profession, maybe 5 or 10 percent, can act in an abrupt way in order to reestablish their sense of control and say things like "No patient of mine is going to become an addict. I'm only going to give you so much medicine," but, interestingly, this desire for control can swing the other way, and the physician can say, "No patient of mine is going to experience any discomfort," and then they give the patient an overdose. That has happened, too, here in Oregon. Patients have been given an overdose to reestablish the doctor's control, in my view, rather than really work with the patient on controlling their pain. These doctors don't eliminate the pain, they eliminate the patient. There are great programs educating physicians how to manage pain and also how to manage their own feelings. The AMA puts some on, my organization puts some on. We don't want doctors to panic and do something untoward, like refuse needed medication or kill the patient.

Is it your experience that stoicism has deep roots in our culture?
Actually, stoicism has been eliminated from our culture in the last twenty years. I don't think you're going to find many stoics around. You're going to find a lot of hedonists—people who really think that pleasure is what makes life meaningful. (*laughing*) People think they should be happy. People think they have a right to be happy. People have a hard time finding meaning in doing things that are difficult, perhaps even painful. Not everybody, but many people almost worship happiness and pleasure.

I wonder if there is a link between a disdain for hedonism and the fact that we seem generally more concerned that people not abuse drugs than that they live free from unnecessary chronic pain.
There is a great fear of drug abuse, and rightly so. We have a very, very high addiction rate in this culture. Addiction is a very serious problem. It can ruin lives. To treat it, you need both a regulatory and a caring component. You have to say that it's wrong and you want it to stop, and that to accomplish that you're going to do this, that, and the other thing; but you also have to understand that addiction is a biological problem with a strong genetic component. When people become addicts they are still good people, and you

have to fight the addiction, not the person. Some employers do this. They say if you don't stop this, you're going to lose your job, but if you follow a program, then you get to keep your job. It's the same thing with marriages, legal troubles, driving drunk, and so on.

While it is right for people to be concerned with addiction, they need to be concerned about chronic pain and suffering, too. I don't think that it's a fear of addiction that keeps physicians from prescribing opioids appropriately—they understand the difference between addiction and physical dependence—but there are people who come in and lie in order to get medicine they don't need. Being aware of those people and their problems and also being concerned with treating chronic pain patients, that's a struggle. Society doesn't like struggles. The media doesn't like struggles. It's easier to put a quota on long-acting opioids than deal with the problem properly. But depriving people in pain of needed medication is a terrible thing to do.

The problem of pain control and the problem of addiction are two entirely different problems in two entirely different patient populations. There really isn't much overlap. If a patient is in serious pain, from cancer for example, you need to forget that they may become physically dependent and treat their pain. Manipulative abusers are a different group with a different problem. People need to understand the difference between addiction and physical dependence and know that these are different problems in different groups of people. Doctors need to know that, too, and to be taught how to treat both groups.

The state of Oregon limits how much pain medicine can be given to a patient. Although it's a particularly appalling example, it isn't the first time good medicine and tight budgets have tangled. What's your take on this issue?

Oregon has the Oregon Health Plan, the only rationed state health care plan in the country. In 1998, that plan put an arbitrary cap on the amount of some of the best long-acting opioid pain medicines that doctors could obtain for their patients without obtaining permission that was nearly always denied. In doing so, the state claimed to be following the manufacturer's guidelines, but when my group called the manufacturer, we learned those were not their guidelines at all. Then the state contended that the cap was for medical reasons. We looked into that and found that there were no medical reasons. Because the body develops a tolerance to opioids, limiting dosage doesn't work. There is no upper dose limit. The state's limit was inadequate. Patients were suffering and doctors couldn't help them because the state had set up multiple hoops for the doctor to jump through. Even when the doctor wrote the prescriptions, the patients couldn't get the medicines paid for. That was a terrible thing, and it happened within a few months of the Plan fully funding assisted suicide. So here these poor patients couldn't get their pain medicine, but they could get a fully-funded death.

To make matters worse, the Plan is now concocting a formulary based on price, so that doctors will have to use the cheapest, rather than the best drugs. Health care should be between the doctor and the patient, not the state. This issue is rearing its ugly head on a national basis now, not because of a limit on the amounts of opioid that can be prescribed, but on the amount of opioids that can be manufactured! Incomprehensible! Ludicrous!

How did you become involved in all this?

Until the assisted-suicide movement here in Oregon, as well as the controversy over pain care, I had what you might call a fairly refined and somewhat sedate practice. But I was morally obliged to step forward and say publicly that we can treat pain and we can treat depression and we can alleviate suffering, and we don't have to kill our patients to do it.

Marcia Gill, R.N.,
M.H.M, C.H.T.P.

৩৩

Marcia Gill is the former director of the John W. Henry Center for Integrative Medicine at Boca Raton Community Hospital, a registered nurse, and a healing touch practitioner. I interview her at the center in South Florida.

How have your experiences with healing touch enhanced your understanding of pain and the human body?

When I learned about pain in nursing school, it was about the physiological process of pain, and maybe some of the emotional aspects. Nowadays I see pain as having multiple causes, and as being a manifestation of an imbalance in the body's energy system. Healing touch focuses on the chakras, and the energy fields that surround the body. In traditional Western medicine we try to look for the cause and treat it—medicate for it. But a patient is the union of body mind and spirit, and as a result, pain can be sensed in the body's energy field, usually over the areas of the body where it is experienced. To go at pain internally with medication is often necessary, because if someone is in acute pain they are not going to lie still for a healing touch session, but the pain needs to be dealt with on other levels, energetically, psychosocially, and so on.

Migraine headaches are a good example. When someone is having a migraine, or has recently had one, there's a clear energy spike. It's palpable many feet away. In healing touch we generally scan the area with our hands. When you pass through that spike, the person flinches. You keep going in and out, unruffling and unruffling and unruffling until the patient can't feel you anymore and you can be ten feet out and still feel the spike. It's the most amazing thing I've ever seen, and the most dramatic example of pain manifesting itself energetically. So when you do an energetic assessment with the hands—there are some people, by the way, who have the visual ability to see the energy fields, although personally I can't do this—the hands intuitively, kinesthetically, know where to go. Energy is a component to pain that isn't generally addressed unless the person is routinely experiencing energy medicine.

Some patients complain that when a clear physical cause of their distress is not immediately evident, they are disbelieved. Do you think there is a parallel disbelief in a healing system that does not reveal itself to the everyday tools of Western medicine?

I suppose there is. Someone who will not accept the possibility that anything outside their immediate scope of learning exists will probably have a closed mind toward both inexplicable pain and a therapeutic modality that can't be put under a microscope. Most of my life has been spent in oncology. A high percentage of an oncologist's patients end up succumbing to their disease. Even though they are unlikely to recommend an alternative therapy, most oncologists are supportive of a patient's desire to try something different. I have not come face-to-face with the rigid dismissal that some doctors may exhibit, saying this stuff is all nonsense, that it doesn't exist.

Sometimes, experiences with patients open the door for the doctors themselves. When I went to my first healing-touch

workshop and heard the lecturer talking about chakras and energy fields, I thought I had never heard such bull in all my life. I
completely disbelieved that anything like that could exist, because I'd never heard of it. I was still young enough then to think
that I knew a lot, but over the next few years I had different experiences and that door opened for me. I started reading in areas
that I never knew existed, and then I was reintroduced to the
same material, the same philosophy, and saw it through different
eyes. Now it's clear to me that there is more than we can touch
and feel. The older you get the more you realize how much there
is out there and how little you actually know.

When a patient complains to you about pain, what is your first reaction?
I try to attend to the person, to open my heart to them. I try to
sit with full attention and notice their body language. You can
learn a lot from the way people shift and move and whether or
not they can look you in the eye. Back in 1984 I had surgery and
I received technically great care, but in the five days I was in the
hospital, I could count on the fingers of one hand the number of
times anyone actually looked directly at me and was fully present
for me. Attention is necessary. It's what starts the healing
process. Many people who go to physicians come away feeling
dissatisfied, feeling they haven't been fully listened to.

By paying full attention, do you mean bearing witness to suffering?
That sounds too detached to me. A witness can be someone who
is paying full attention, but as a term it lacks engagement. The
patient needs to feel that you are involved. Sometimes it's hard to
give that. A nurse on a hospital floor, for example, has so much to
remember that while she is doing one thing for one patient she is
thinking about what she has to do for the next. Very often the
patient doesn't feel as if they have her full attention.

Compassion, engagement, is a recurring theme in this book. There seems to be quite a lack of it, both from the patient's perspective and from the health caregiver's, too. Do you have a sense of why that might be?

The stress on caregivers is enormous. The day gets away from you. Even in this center, which is supposed to be a nurturing environment, there are many stresses. In a medical practice where a certain number of patients need to be seen in a set period of time and there are countless unexpected interruptions, keeping to a schedule is tough and the pressure is even higher.

Why do you suppose it is that our culture puts so many things ahead of care and caring?

There's a premium in our modern world on being successful.

Do you mean in a material way?

In a material way, yes. Being busy. Always doing. Our yoga teacher here at the center says we are human beings, not human doings. That's a wonderful phrase. I'm amazed that even little children in primary grades have such full schedules. You've seen the ad on TV where the father has to make an appointment with his kid? I believe it started when we lost Sundays. We used to keep the Sabbath, on whatever day. We used to have a day of rest in our religious traditions, a day for religious ritual and tradition, a time for family, a day separate from the other six days of the week. It was an opportunity to wind down, to come back to baseline, to come back to normal before your week started off again. When stores started opening on Sundays, people became busier, more active, and they lost that opportunity to regain homeostasis, to regain our balance. We're like hamsters on a treadmill now. We're in perpetual motion. This frenzy has carried over into how we treat others. We have forgotten how to listen, and how to be fully, mindfully present for the person you are with at the moment that you're with them.

We've explored the premium placed on being busy. Do you think there may also be a premium placed on enduring pain, on suffering?

I think that premium exists but that it predates the condition we find ourselves in our culture. The notion that suffering redeems us, that it is, to some extent, good for us, comes from our religious values. Suffering builds character. It helps to expiate your time in purgatory. Also, there's a benefit to being able to take a bit of pain and suffering, because we're going to experience it in daily life, if only as the crick in the neck we wake up with as we get older. But people who are in severe pain, like the pain of metastatic disease or trauma, are seen differently, although all of us have different pain thresholds and different wiring. To impose your experience on someone else is inappropriate. Culturally we see differences in the way people respond to pain. Northern Europeans tend to be more stoic, whereas Mediterranean people tend to be more expressive. Last night on the news I saw a story about one young man here in South Florida, an immigrant from the Caribbean, who shot another over a bicycle. There was great weeping and wailing and the throwing up of hands in the air and falling. That's the way their culture shows grief. Contrast that with Jacqueline Kennedy. How you are brought up to deal with pain has a lot to do with how you experience it. It's very complex.

Besides pain medications, surgery, physical therapy and healing touch, what techniques do you think are helpful?

Relaxation techniques. Meditation. Breathing. All those help change the perception of pain and may also relieve it directly because pain can be associated with muscle tension, with tightening up. Learning to relax and breathing into the pain, even though it's hard to do at first because people want to block the experience, often lessens the pain. What's important to remember is that we all heal ourselves. Doctors don't heal us; they just give us the tools to do it. We've abrogated that responsibility. We have delegated it to others. That may be one of the pressures that physicians feel. They may feel somehow impelled to fix everything that comes to them, and very often they don't know how. Very often people will call this center and say, "I have this condition and that condition. What can you do for me?" Right away we feel, "Wow, I really have to come up with something for that person."

And the patient's question really should be "What can I do for myself and how can you help me?"

Exactly.

Ronald Melzack, Ph.D.

ꙮ

Dr. Ronald Melzack is one of the seminal thinkers in the field of pain. Cofounder of McGill University's pain center and author of the now-ubiquitous McGill Pain Questionnaire, his awards and publications—which include the Order of Canada, countless groundbreaking studies in juried professional journals, and editorship of the gold-standard "Textbook of Pain"—are too numerous to list. He is also the author of four celebrated children's books. I interview him at his office in Montreal, Quebec.

Tell me how you came to explore pain.

I'm a psychologist. I got my Ph.D. here at McGill with a remarkable man called Donald Hebb, who really was the founder of contemporary cognitive psychology. In the course of working toward my Ph.D., I was searching for a topic for my thesis and came across the problem of pain in a study on Scottish terriers that was being done in Hebb's laboratory. The dogs were raised in cages in which their environment was restricted to the cage itself. They had a clean cage and lots of food every day, but no opportunity to see or hear much, and none in which they ever fought with each other, as there was only one dog to a cage. They lived that way until they were six months old.

When they came out, the terriers seemed not to respond to pain appropriately. If I lit a match they would run over and stick their nose into the match. What that study showed was that there was learning involved in pain, that we have to discover that something hurts us or does not hurt us. The fact that past experience gives our pain perceptions meaning was recognized for the first time in that trial.

You called pain a "problem." Can you elaborate on that?

This work took place in the 1950s, when we thought that pain was virtually defined as the response to a physical injury. Back then there was little distinction between the experience of pain and the mechanisms of pain, although I was convinced that there was more to it. Other people were thinking that way too, but our ideas didn't fit into any conceptual framework at that time. There was a fellow called Beecher, an anesthesiologist, who received men who had been wounded in battle at the Anzio beachhead. He found that three out of four of these guys would say that they were not in pain. He was also the one who looked at the placebo effect, which he suggested was obviously very important in whether or not we perceive an injury as being painful. So I thought I had gotten into a very interesting field, although there were very few people working in it back then, perhaps a dozen worldwide.

Amazing, considering how pain is such an important part of life.

That's right. Anyway, the terrier study became my Ph.D. thesis, and I became fascinated with the field. I decided that I needed to discover more about the brain and how it worked, and found out that an important surgeon out in Portland, Oregon, a man called William Livingston, was very interested in pain after relatively minor nerve injuries, and in so-called phantom limb pain. He had started a pain clinic, and had a small, active pain laboratory. I applied and got a fellowship to work with him for one year and ended up working with him for three. They were tremendously important years in my career.

In the first year we mapped pain pathways, trying to figure out where signals go in the brain. We found that after an injury occurred there was not one pain pathway, but five, with evidence that there were a couple more. They streamed to all parts of the brain, not just going from injury point A to brain point B. Then Livingston did a wonderful thing. He said, "Ron, if you're going to learn about pain, you have to come see patients who are experiencing it." With that he invited me to come join his pain clinic, just to come every Tuesday when patients with difficult pain problems were treated. I started to attend those pain clinics and a little seminar in which people would talk about the problem of pain, and began to realize that pain was something you subjectively *feel*.

That was the first time I encountered someone with phantom-limb pain. She was a woman in her seventies, a diabetic who developed gangrene in her foot. Her leg had to be amputated, and subsequently, the other leg did also. She had a very rich vocabulary, and I began to write down the words that she used to describe her pain. I collected these words, and began to add to them words from other patients and from articles I read. I came up with about 150 words. Later, in 1959, I got an appointment as an assistant professor at Massachusetts Institute of Technology. I met a superb statistician there named Warren Torgerson, and together we did work on the language of pain. We wrote a research paper, using his complex statistical methods and the language I had collected. Out of that came a tool to measure pain called the McGill Pain Questionnaire, which has been translated into virtually every language and is now the most widely used questionnaire of its kind in the world.

Do you remember some of the more interesting words people used?
"Burning," "shooting," "stabbing," "wrenching," "crushing." These are how people described a phantom foot, one that had been cut

off and was no longer there, as being in a vice, and the vice was being turned and the foot was being crushed, and all the while, of course, they had no foot. Or they said that there was a red-hot poker being shoved through their ankle, in one side and out the other, and it hurt like hell. And there was no foot, no ankle, nothing below a stump at knee or crotch level. I remember one of my Ph.D. students interviewing an amputee and staring at where the missing foot would be while the patient convincingly described the pain it was giving her. All of us working with phantomlimb pain have experiences like that.

If you can so acutely feel things that are not there, what happens if you pursue the phenomenon to its logical conclusion, hypothetically vivisecting until there's nothing left but the head, and then even further, chopping away at the parts of the brain that are not relevant to this process? Don't you end up questioning the nature of physical reality and bumping up against a spiritual notion of the self?

You do, and I have. I have proposed that there is a complex neural network in the brain, which I call the "neuromatrix." There are a number of these neuromatrices, one of them is for the body-self. Built into this structure is the capacity to feel perceptual features, such as stabbing, hot-burning, and emotional aspects, which suggests that limbic structures are involved, as well as cognitive aspects, such as—What is the meaning of this pain I'm feeling? Did I eat too much last night or do I have cancer? If you took a person's brain, put it in a robot like R2D2 in *Star Wars*, that brain would feel a body, might even feel pain in that body. You do not need a body to feel a body. I keep saying this about pain, and people keep quoting it, but it's true for *all* of our perceptions and all our thoughts. I've done studies, as have others, of people who were born without limbs altogether and have phantom limbs. That literature is growing.

So the brain has a sense of what the body should be.

Absolutely. The brain knows that there are supposed to be arms and legs. It is born with that knowledge.

If there can be no body and you can still have pain, isn't that the ultimate statement of pain's purely experiential nature?

Absolutely. And it tells you how complicated pain must be and how complicated our perception of the body must be.

It also suggests that myriad factors that don't have anything to do with a physical diagnosis, and are therefore so often ignored during treatment, must actually be critically important.

Exactly. That's why it is so difficult to treat pain, and that's why we are just beginning to recognize the importance of drugs that have an effect of disconduction in the nervous system, apart from blocking pain signals—drugs that have an effect on brain activities such as emotions and motivations. That's why some of the best drugs for chronic pain, even cancer pain, are antidepressants and anti-epilepsy drugs. It is all beginning to fall into place.

I see a Buddha behind your desk, and an acupuncture model, too. Have you made a connection between your studies and the Buddhist ideas of pain and suffering?

I've read quite a bit about the Buddhist notions of pain. Those ideas are right. What we are saying now comes very close to Buddhism. How you get those ideas across to a whole lot of people who are contemplating the nature of life and the role of pain in it, that's something perhaps you can achieve with your book.

Acupuncture deals with structures that one could liken to a phantom limb, at least in the sense that you can't see them but they seem to be there. Does acupuncture's effectiveness evoke your neuromatrix?

Acupuncture could produce a sensory input that activates mechanisms in the brain that inhibit sensory input through the spinal cord. I recently read a very good review of the literature on acupuncture and pain. The sad story is that there have not been very good studies. This isn't because people who do acupuncture don't want them, but because it is very easy to get a placebo effect. That effect is so powerful that if you really want to rule it out you have to be able to set a baseline, and the nature of acupuncture makes that hard to do. The authors were Scandinavian rheumatologists who were very sympathetic to acupuncture's effectiveness, but they found the literature wobbly. Maybe the needles release endorphins, but we don't really know.

Is it hard to convey the neuromatrix concept to physicians whose training is very grounded in nuts-and-bolts medicine?

My whole career has been about trying to get my colleagues to understand what I'm trying to say. I have a better chance with folks who *don't* have medical training, who haven't studied spinal cord physiology. Some of my most impressive colleagues, folks who win tremendous awards and huge research grants, are comfortable with the spinal cord. They like an input/output system. That's what they need. I had an easier time, with my friend and colleague Patrick Wall, propounding our gate-control theory than the neuromatrix.

What is the "gate-control theory"?

It says that there are gating mechanisms in the dorsal horns of the spinal cord. These gates can open and close, a matter of inhibition or excitation, to allow information to pass through or to block it out. So if you're a football player and you get a kick in the shin and your shin bone cracks, you might not feel it at all because you are busy looking at something else and your brain shuts the gates. On the other hand, if you think a bloated feeling in your guts after a big meal might mean cancer, gates open wide and you feel pain.

I'm interested in the notion that physicians are so steeped in the mechanics of the biological process that they find your theoretical model of pain difficult to accept. Is there no way to show them something concrete, something they can see?

When people were first talking about genes, no one had seen a gene.

And we were able to vaporize Hiroshima without seeing an atom.

Exactly. Some of my colleagues don't believe the neuromatrix is a useful concept because they can't get into the brain and see it. They say, "Forget about the brain. We're looking at the spinal cord, at inflammation in the skin. We're looking at transmitters at synapses." Now, I've received all the honors I can from my colleagues in Canada, and they know I've made important contributions with the gate theory and with the McGill Pain Questionnaire, but the neuromatrix idea worries them. A friend stated it very well in a letter to me. He said, "Ron, you're right. Of course pain is in the brain. But to get my research grants, I have to go to a committee that knows how to do rigid, straightforward experiments on the spinal cord. I want to get grants, so therefore I'm going to stick with the spinal cord."

What's unacceptable about that is that the flow of money and the vicissitudes of politics leave people in pain to pay the price.

You're right, of course. The good news is that there are there are plenty of ways to get at something without seeing it, and there are new generations of doctors, students, physiologists and pharmacologists, who are, to my astonishment, increasingly open to my ideas. Often the term "neuromatrix" isn't even attributed to me and I don't care. It's a joy just to see it in the literature. They think the McGill Pain Questionnaire was made up by some guy named McGill. I don't care about that either. I'm just glad it's being used. The pain a person feels is made up of not only the disease processes going on in the body but that person's hopes and expectations for himself and his children. It is determined by past generations, by fears and anxieties, by all the activities in which the brain is involved.

My sister's husband died a terrible death because people have stupid ideas about tolerance and addiction, stupid ideas about how—if you gave opioid medications too soon—they wouldn't work when the person needed them more urgently. We now know that was all nonsense, but poor Harry died in agony anyway. I wrote an article on the tragedy of needless pain for *Scientific American* and became very interested in opioids and their actions. I did quite a bit of research about them, and am now editing a textbook of pain and a handbook of pain management. The most important chapters in that book are the chapters on cancer pain and other severe chronic pain. Palliative-care units now use pain questionnaires and use drugs more appropriately; they decrease anxiety and they mitigate suffering. That's what really counts. Using knowledge compassionately. It's all about compassion.

PART THREE

Thinkers About Pain

L IKE ELECTRICITY, MAGNETISM, RADIOWAVES, AND
sonar, pain exists even though it cannot always be seen. Clergy
and counselors, ethicists and philosophers have all paid a great deal
of attention to it because it is a centerpiece of the human condition.
But our religious views may insidiously lead to preconceptions and
prejudices where pain is concerned, and in important ways the
mental and the spiritual aspects of pain remain as poorly understood as atomic energy was in the early days. Pain is related to
death, and, therefore, has a link to hell, to retribution, comeup-
pance, karma, punishment, Judgment Day, and to the perceived
value of a human being.

A romance with stoicism, traceable back far beyond our Puritan
roots, pervades our culture, even to the point where pain is considered a critical, if not an essential part of art. A basic tenet of every
form of artistic expression is that there must be conflict, angst, trial,
overcoming, triumph, and resolution. The characters that artists
render—whether on the big screen, the small screen, the stage, on
canvas, or between the pages of a book—must feel pain as we do,
sometimes to a seemingly unendurable degree, in order to affect us
as art should. Pain authenticates life the same way it authenticates art.

When it comes right down to it, there is an implication in the way most of us look at pain that we are most keenly alive when we are feeling either the greatest pleasure or the greatest pain. Religiously, philosophically, ethically, we are still after the truth about pain.

The same is true in medicine. Though great progress has indisputably been made—doctors did not used to put people to sleep for amputations, holding them down instead while they sawed off offending limbs—there is still much work to be done. As recently as fifteen years ago doctors were performing surgery on infants without anesthesia, using only paralytic agents to make sure they didn't move. Many circumcisions are still performed without anesthesia, even though tests now show that fetuses as young as twenty three weeks respond to painful stimuli. Doctors now know that pain interferes with recovery; that it hampers an organism's ability to heal; that it brings with it direct physical consequences, such as increased blood pressure and resulting stroke, heart attack, seizure, or brain hemorrhage. Medical researchers have also discovered that untreated pain has the sort of emotional consequences—fears, phobias, delayed defensive reactions and sensitivities—in test animals that make one wonder whether the brutalities until recently visited on infants might later in life lead to violent or sociopathic behavior, or a predilection toward substance abuse.

The adaptive value of pain has been extensively investigated, as has its biological purpose—the role it serves in letting us know not to stick our finger in the fire, not to eat those habañero peppers again, not to lift another heavy sack without bending our knees. The distinction between the message of acute pain and the pathological persistence of chronic pain, however, has not been studied as deeply. As a result of the Descartian split between the mind and the body—a split that implies that there is something less lofty, less God-like, less quintessentially *human* about the body than there is about the mind—pain has, in the past, been deconstructed into emotional and physical form. Because of the recent recognition of therapies such as hypnosis and acupuncture, and because of new medical models that show that pain is far more a function of the brain and the spinal cord than of the peripheral nerves, mind and body elements have been reintegrated. This joining has spawned what is known as mind/body medicine: a field that has been in existence in the East for millennia simply as "medicine."

Much of recent medical work has been important and helpful, but some of it may have been conducted in much the way a savant multiplies columns of numbers or calculates the odds in a poker game—without a guiding conscience. Exploration of biological phenomena—without the appropriate moral and spiritual context—can lead to excrescences, such as the "work" of Josef Mengele or the Marquis de Sade. Like other branches of science, medicine has long eschewed basing conclusions and decisions on emotion—fearing it so much that some doctors would rather avoid common sense and risk causing their patients agony than be thought to be anything but objective, dispassionate, and correct. The trouble is that the practice of medicine is not a field of basic inquiry, but a field of service. Its purpose is not to generate hypotheses and tests, but to heal. Without compassion, medicine is devoid of its *raison d'être*.

Consider, too, the role of the war on drugs on compassionate, effective pain management. Although quality of life has become a hot topic, and the undertreatment of pain by a doctor a legally actionable offense, opioid analgesics, the most potent pain medicines in a doctor's arsenal, are limited, controlled, and even shunned because they may be abused by drug abusers. Many chronic pain patients will not admit to needing more pain medication even when they do, because they fear addiction more than suffering. Medications that are part of the solution in the war against chronic pain have become part of the problem in a campaign driven by a government more comfortable with addressing law-enforcement challenges than social ones. Drug diversion and black-market profiteering make the problem worse; a few bad apples spoil it for those in genuine need. The fact that better pain management does not lead to more addicts is often overlooked.

Finally, we cannot ignore the lack of compassion endemic to a health care system where profit rather than outcome is the guiding principle. Despite modern medicine's ability to ease or even banish it, pain persists because proper pain management often cannot be accomplished in the brief visits allowed by managed care. Worse, many prescription plans and health insurance policies put a cap on how much pain medication patients may receive, leaving people to live on in agony after the policy limit is reached. It is more than possible that the economic model of health care and thorough pain management are antithetical.

The thinkers who hold forth in this final section of the book address these tangled dimensions of pain. There are a number of viewpoints here, with some emphasis on the Buddhist perspective—Buddhism has wise and important things to say about suffering and compassion—but all coming to the consensus that it is time for a change in the way we think about chronic pain and suffering.

June Dahl, Ph.D.

~

Dr. June Dahl is a professor of pharmacology at the University of Wisconsin, Madison. Her work as one of the architects of the Wisconsin Cancer Pain Initiative has contributed greatly to the national forum on the undertreatment of pain. I interview her in New York City.

Why do you suppose that only a certain percentage of those who suffer an injury or disease become chronic pain patients?

I wish I knew the answer to that question. It is possible that there is something physiologically different about people who go on to develop chronic pain syndrome. It could be some difference in the makeup of their spinal cords that results in differential changes in those parts of the spinal cord that respond to noxious stimuli like pain, but we don't really know. What's exciting in today's world is that there are so many advances in our understanding of pain mechanisms and processes that maybe the answer to your very difficult question will soon emerge.

Do you think that there is a personality type that is more likely to become a chronic pain patient?

I don't have any evidence to say yes or no to your question, and since my background is in science, I don't like to render opinions without evidence. Sometimes I think there might be something of that sort, but on the other hand we have to reflect on the changes that occur in personality and behavior because people have a persistent pain problem. So which comes first? It's that old proverbial chicken or egg question.

191

Tell me about the Wisconsin Cancer Pain Initiative.

In essence the Pain Initiative is an advocacy and educational organization, a grassroots volunteer organization of health care professionals. It was formed to confront the barriers that have been identified as being responsible for the undertreatment of pain. When it
began back in 1986, and was named a demonstration project of the
World Health Organization, it was a lone voice crying in the
wilderness. There were at that time no national efforts dedicated to
improving pain management. It wasn't until the 1990s that we
began to see the Oncology Nursing Society, the National Cancer
Institute, and now, finally, the American Cancer Society, recognize
the under-treatment of pain as a major public health problem and
begin to develop strategies to deal with it. The initiative's mission
is very straightforward, namely to address the lack of knowledge
and inappropriate attitudes of health care professionals, patients,
and families, and to address regulatory barriers and barriers in the
health care system. That includes barriers in the reimbursement
system, in the way we pay for health care in this country, and in the
context of that, appreciating that so many people have no insurance and no way to pay for expensive pain medicines.

What has working with the Initiative taught you?

That you can educate and advocate a great deal and still not get
at the persistent barriers in the health care system responsible for
the undertreatment of pain that helped lead to measurable
change. In September 1996, the American Cancer Society held a
pain summit. Lots of people came to try and develop more
strategies to deal with the pain of cancer. I was cochair of a panel
charged with drafting strategies to change physician practice. We
sat around for an hour or so and finally agreed on what we already knew, namely that education does not change behavior.
You have to make changes in the system itself, in the institutions
in which people practice, in order to bring lasting change.

Have your colleagues ever frustrated you?

All of us who work in the area of pain management have been frustrated with colleagues who don't seem to realize how much people suffer and how much unrelieved pain changes lives. Sometimes you feel that the only way you can make them understand is to throw them off a cliff and break all their bones. I recall a physician who was interviewed by a national medical journal upon the occasion of his retirement. He said that now that he had reached the end of his career, he had great regret about one thing, and that was that he had not, in all of his practice time, really understood how much his patients were suffering, and that he had not addressed their pain adequately. The realization came from the fact that shortly after he retired, he was hospitalized with a serious medical problem that required major surgery and his pain was not well managed. He could not convince his colleagues that he hurt so much that they needed to do something.

Sometimes it takes that kind of personal experience to really understand. Not always, but sometimes. I used to team teach with the director of our student health services, who would say to the medical students, when he talked about pain management and doses of drugs, "Give as you would receive." The students would look at him with total blank stares, because when you are a young doc, you just generally never have had any significant pain problems, nor even had a family member who has had a serious disease and experienced serious pain.

But compassion is not enough.

No, compassion is not enough. It's very important to be *passionate* about what you do, and in the context of being passionate, you certainly develop compassion for individuals, but you cannot provide relief with compassion alone. You have to couple it with really significant knowledge and skills about how to address specific pain problems using the therapies that are available. When we started the WCPI, one of the basic principles that we were operating on was that we knew how to manage pain. The problem wasn't the lack of therapies. The problem was that those therapies were not being used appropriately.

Would you be surprised to hear that the preponderance of pain patients I have interviewed have cited the lack of physician compassion as a greater problem than the lack of physician competence?

No, I wouldn't be surprised that patients sense that lack of compassion. It's easy to indict the medical profession. But we also have to recognize the basic principles of the health care system in this country. We operate on an acute-care model. The thrust in American medicine has been to cut and to cure. The caring component has been left out. Physicians really feel that they have to do everything they can to make people well. In the process of that they forget about controlling the symptoms that may be destroying the quality of a patient's life.

The system may indeed be flawed in terms of its politics, sensitivities, and the financial model it obeys, but my guess is that the physician as mechanic, as fixer, is a concept that doesn't spring from our health care system, but rather the reverse.

I agree. But let's be practical about things. We say that if only the doctor would assess and treat pain properly everything would be just fine, and certainly there are circumstances in which physicians may not know how to treat pain or be sensitive to their patients' needs, but the demands on physicians' time in today's world are incredible. On top of that, technological and pharmacological advances are saving patients who would have died as recently as ten or fifteen years ago, so there are new medical challenges for the doctor, not to mention pressure from third-party payers, which limit the amount of time they can spend with patients. It is easy to castigate physicians for their presumed lack of caring, but we have to think more broadly about the issues that exist in our society, and particularly about the way we deliver health care. We take care of the wealthy very well, but we don't seem to have much concern about those without the financial resources to pay. I deplore the fact that we don't have a universal health care system.

It has never been my intention to cast aspersions on the personal character of physicians. Even if the system we have today arose from the model of doctor as mechanic, today's physicians were not there when that happened and are not to blame for it. It may be, however, that their strong efforts are required to help us change it.

If you look at the way physicians are trained today, the model is extraordinarily inhumane. The demands that are put on residents, for example, can really put patients at jeopardy.

It can really put the residents themselves in jeopardy, too, physically, from sleep deprivation, and legally and emotionally, from mistakes they might make.

Absolutely. And there are many people who have lobbied for serious change and written about it in august medical journals. But boy, that is a tough nut to crack. I don't know how you are going to break into that tradition. The folks who are practicing now say, "Well, I went through it. You can, too."

I saw this in my own veterinary medical training.

It's a human tragedy of enormous dimension. You are so right when you point out that there is more than just an adverse effect on patient care. You have to think of the adverse affects on the humans who are providing care, because in the process of this training, they can often lose a lot of their humanity. They go to medical school all bright-eyed and bushy-tailed, wanting to save the world. . . .

And they come out cynical, exhausted and jaded.

You've got the words. And it's *so* sad. I see these kids when they come into school and they are good people who want to do everything they can to take care of people who are sick.

The stoicism that is required of medical students during the hazing process that is their medical training reminds me of the stoicism some physicians expect from patients in chronic pain.

We still have a lot of Puritan tradition within us.

I didn't necessarily mean that there was a cause-and-effect relationship, but rather that both are a manifestation of a larger problem.

I agree. I come out of a strange, small-town midwestern culture, a Calvinist tradition that says that doing anything to feel good is bad.

What is that all about?

Life is serious. You're supposed to work all the time and never have fun.

Big mistake.

I know it is. But when you come out of such a background, it's hard to understand some cultures—the tremendous fun-loving warmth of Italians, for example. I envy them so much! But when you're in this puritanical Northern European mode, it is sometimes hard to transform into a fun-loving free spirit.

Do you think that such a prejudice against pleasure has anything to do with the prejudices against drug addiction?

Boy, I really do think there's a relationship. When you look at chapters on opioid analgesics in old medical textbooks, you wouldn't find a title such as "Morphine and Other Wonderful Substances." In fact, you would find titles such as "Morphine and Other Addicting Drugs." When you think of the effects of opioids, they are great analgesics that make people feel good. That doesn't mean that they create euphoria, but that *by taking the pain away you make the patient feel better.* Somehow that seems inappropriate in a Puritanical culture.

This prejudice against feeling good is evident not only amongst some health care providers, but also in pain patients and their families.
True. If you look back on the history of our attitudes about pain and pain medicine in this country, you will find a lot of confusion. Surgeons used to think that pain was essential to healing. That was a prevalent perspective in the 1800s.

Not that long ago.
That's right. But because medicine is such a traditional profession, even perspectives that were held fifty years ago may still pervade individuals working inside the system. Also, there has been so much confusion about the medicines because after the Harrison Narcotic Act, we began to persecute, de-license, and jail physicians who were maintaining patients on opioids. That created an attitude that physicians were the cause of addiction. It is confusing to physicians that we have pain patients who are using opioids to cope with circumstances in their lives. That is absolutely against the law and against medical practice.

But what about antidepressants?
There are people who are critical of those, too. But nothing is held in more disfavor than abusing a controlled substance.

When you say "controlled," I have to ask "controlled by whom"? Not by God, certainly, but by laws passed by our own representatives.
One of the important jobs of the WCPI is to engage governmental authorities who are passing regulations that impede access to drugs and make crazy statements such as "It's okay to provide an opioid to someone who has advanced disease, even if it hastens death." There is no evidence for anything like that. It's a myth. A myth in law. The myth of double effect.

*So what would hasten death, in fact, would be to perform surgery with-
out anesthesia, as used to be common practice, but not to make a patient
more comfortable.*

Most hospice people will tell you that aggressive pain management probably prolongs life. Sometimes when family members
call me because their loved ones won't take their medicine because they are afraid of becoming addicted to it, I'll say to the
family member, "Look. *Pain is bad for you.* There is evidence that
your loved one will live longer if they take their medication."
Somehow there is this perception that pain is a good thing, that
it builds character. I don't see that pain has any redeeming virtues
whatsoever. It destroys character.

I wish that we would not talk about patients' *complaints*, but
rather say that patients *report* a certain intensity or quality of pain.
Complain is the verb we associate with pain, and that seems a very
judgmental description. Medicine tends to be that way. There has
always been a sense that patients are not equal to the doctor. Patients are not accepting that attitude any longer. The Internet is
creating an interesting challenge for physicians. It is so full of truth
and falsehood. People come into the office and challenge their
physicians. I tell my medical students that they had better know
what their patients are reading before they come to you. Some of it
is absolute garbage, of course, but some of it is extremely valuable
and empowers patients to have a learned, constructive dialogue
with their physicians. The really outstanding physicians whom I
know respect their patients for the knowledge they have, and for
taking the time to learn about their problem. Part of the thing with
pain is that if you are ignorant of the facts, if you lack knowledge,
you become fearful and anxious and that makes your pain worse.
Taking the mystery out of pain helps patients cope with it.

Marilyn Vos Savant

ꙮ

Widely appreciated as "the smartest woman in the world," author, thinker, and commentator Marilyn Vos Savant has an audience of 70 million readers every week in her Parade *magazine column, and countless others in her self-help books about the power of reason and logical thinking. I interview Ms. Vos Savant at her New York City penthouse office, overlooking the city's newly bereft landscape.*

Why do you suppose so many people in our society suffer unnecessary physical agony?

I didn't quite realize that the problem was of such magnitude. Within the sector you've described, I would see two types: those who are unable to do anything to relieve their pain no matter how hard they try, and those who are being denied access to treatment. I don't know which is the bigger group. One would presume it is the former, but our conversations lead me to believe it may be the latter. We have a lot of people who are unable to speak for themselves. I think of my grandmother as she lay dying of cancer, for example. I also think of the kind of person who has chronic pain, back pain, say, terrible migraines—people who can't get relief and are branching out into alternative therapies. Which group are we talking about?

Both.

I know a lot of people who actually resist treatment. I know people who tell me they won't even take an aspirin. I wonder why, unless, of course, they have something specifically against aspirin, which is not typically their point. It's a sort of stoicism. There are also people afraid of pain medicine, not so much because of fear of addiction, but because they want to keep something in reserve in case the pain gets worse. I had surgery and I felt this way. I always wanted to take things minimally because I had in the back of my mind that if the pain got worse I could always do such and such. Of course, I'm healthy and have never reached the extreme where I was just begging for whatever was available, though I know people do reach that miserable point. I don't know who speaks for them. You would think the doctor would, as his or her advocate.

But doctors seem to be a little bit less like that now. Although I'm not saying anything negative about them—my husband is an M.D. although he doesn't have a traditional practice and, in a lot of ways, I think doctors are saints—but they do have additional concerns now. They are worried about liability. They are worried about doing anything that could get them criticism, and that's understandable. I would feel guilty about implying that doctors would ever withhold pain medication because of concerns about hastening death, in the case of morphine, for example, but doctors may lag a bit in terms of what they *could* do. This may in part be due to the way I felt after surgery—that the doctor is keeping something in reserve. Of course it did occur to me afterwards that the doctor wasn't prescribing anywhere near what I could have had if I had needed it.

Do you think we should be more responsible for our own health care, or continue to do as we have done, namely abdicate it, primarily to medical doctors?

We are 100-percent responsible for our own health, but I don't think we always have the expertise to do what we need. A person lying in a hospital bed, someone just taken out of the World Trade Center, that's one thing, but in my case, obviously I should go and find the expert who knows what I need. So maybe it's a continuum rather than a social issue of how much should we help ourselves or others. In this society, living here in New York, for example, one of the reasons we are so vulnerable is that we are all interdependent. None of us has what it takes to live on our own. The most that I can do, for example, is go and stock up on two weeks worth of food if I didn't want to have to go out. I can't grow my own food. We are all dependent on each other to do our part, our little piece. If we grant that, if we say that the more civilized you get, the further you get from an agrarian economy, the more it's going to be like that.

Let's talk about the agrarian society for a moment. In a village, you have no insurance, and caretaking happens within the family and the super-family. People provide for each other. That clear interdependence is the grease that keeps the gears turning. But as the society becomes more complex, that grease may dry up. It seems that it has dried up in our culture, and I say that because so basic a thing as relief from pain may not be available or may be denied.

I'm wondering what you mean by "denied." It sounds as if you think you have a right to pain relief.

Do you not think that to live as pain free as possible is a right?

No, I don't. I think that it is in conflict with nature. It's too much of an expectation for a human being. It's like asking whether I have a right to as much medical care as I need. That's a tricky one, of course, because I might decide that I need a lot more medical care than someone else thinks I need. Do I have a right to that? Well, someone else has to provide it, so I would be asking other people to be my slaves. It would be enslaving people—not literally enslaving, because one chooses to be a doctor versus a gardener—but it implies that someone somewhere must take care of me. If I extend that to a right to be pain free, insofar as society is able to make that happen, it would seem that pharmaceutical companies, say, would have to provide me with whatever it is I want or need, yet they have to go spend, $400,000,000 or whatever it takes, to get an average new drug through the FDA.

Do you think we have a right to have enough to eat?
Are we speaking of rights as a citizen or rights as a being here on Earth?

I'm responding to the notion that to be pain free is against nature. I'm wondering whether you might say the same thing about having enough to eat, or having shelter over your head.
Gaining that right requires someone to intercede between you and nature. That can happen in the case of food. I'm not sure it can happen in the case of pain. Sometimes it could. It depends upon whether someone is actually being denied relief. I notice you use the word "denied," which you must do for a particular reason. It implies "I'm in pain, I have a right to pain medicine and someone is denying me access." Is that the situation as you see it?

That could be the situation for some people, but let's get back to the food question for a moment. One would not consider farmers or grocery store clerks to be slaves. In the model of an integrated, interdependent society that you advanced earlier, we do things for each other and thereby do things for ourselves. Among the very first things we would do for each other, I would imagine, would be to provide for each other's most basic needs. I tender the opinion that freedom from pain—and I use the word "freedom" loosely—may be our most powerful urge in being alive. I might in fact go so far as to say that life is about seeking pleasure and avoiding pain, although the sources of those things may differ for each of

*us. So I wouldn't agree that people helping others be free of pain were in
any way enslaved.*

Unless it is required.

*I would go back to the questions of food and shelter. Does one have a
right to have enough to eat and have a roof over one's head? Most people would say that those are transcendent rights, that they apply to citizens of the planet Earth or citizens of the United States of America.*

So you are saying that insofar as we have those rights, then we
should also have a right to be free of pain.

Yes. That makes sense.

We are probably quibbling over what we are calling rights. Society certainly provides food, clothing, and shelter to those who
can't manage on their own, although I'm not suggesting we
should be giving out pain medication freely, as we'd be getting
addicts in the street. But insofar as you can say we have rights to
food, clothing, and shelter, it seems reasonable that freedom from
undue pain could be provided. We'd have to come up with a good
definition of "undue" though.

*Most of us have the impulse to help the homeless when we see them,
whether we act on that impulse or not. We also know that there are programs to feed them and get them off the street.*

And we do that for the sick with Medicare and Medicaid. That
should include pain medication, although I'm not saying that is
necessarily enough.

*Why do you suppose the media give much coverage to political ideas and
agendas, and, in a cyclical way, the issues of poverty and starvation, but
not so much to the problem of unrelieved chronic pain?*

It could be because we can't see pain. When someone says they're
hungry, you can know what that feels like. But you can't photo-
graph pain.

So it could be an issue of invisibility?

It could be. And it's difficult to communicate the experience of pain to someone.

Especially so if the pain is chronic. Acute pain, of course, may be the result of visible trauma, a car accident, for example, or there may be hyperventilation, an ashen pallor, sweating, screaming and yelling, and so on. Chronic pain tends to be more occult, and quieter.

We've also become accustomed to people crying wolf about other things. Exaggerating.

If someone complains and you ask them what's wrong and they tell you they're in terrible pain from cancer, you're immediately sympathetic. But if they tell you they just have a sore back or sciatica, it may be harder to know how to respond.

You mention sciatica, which gives this shooting pain. If you've never had that, if you've never been in their shoes for even a moment, you can't know how they feel. Pain ranges all over the place, from sciatica to cluster headaches or burns. It's so varied that it's difficult to understand. There are words that people use to try to describe their pain. It reminds me of the stereotype of the housewife who takes her car to the mechanic and says, "It makes this shushing, pinging sound." Fortunately, a car is fairly simple, so the mechanic knows where to look, but it's different with pain. I wish there were a better way to describe it. I've felt inadequate to that task myself. I wish there were a way to describe pain in colors. That might give us more of a standard. But I suppose there's something like 0–100 and it hurts 90.

There is such a scale.

One of the reasons I mentioned colors is that there is shade, there is hue, there is tone, etc. If we take something obvious, like light blue to royal blue to navy blue, that could be one kind of pain, and then there could be a yellow kind of pain or a red kind of pain, etc. Pain is a qualitative phenomenon, and upsets some people more than others, depending upon what kind of pain it is. I know I've dismissed some pain of my own because I knew what caused it, but if I don't know what it is, it's a lot worse.

You mentioned crying wolf. As a society, I believe we have become desensitized to pain.

Consider the movies! Consider what people tolerate in the movies! Some fellow is shot in the abdomen. . . .

And for a day and a half wanders around in pursuit of a pretty girl.

Ridiculous! (*laughing*) Crazy!

There's a duality, isn't there? On the one hand we're giving a model of Stoicism by larger-than-life heroes on the movie screen, and yet other countries think Americans are soft.

Yes. Consider what's going on in the wake of September 11. People are terrified to go to the mall because something may possibly happen. They're afraid to go across the Golden Gate Bridge because something may possibly happen. I'm not saying that I don't feel discomfort myself. I do. It's disappointing, but we're not in a brave new world at all, we're in a cowardly new world.

Yet, I've found most chronic pain patients to be very brave. Here's this invisible nightmare that they can't communicate and they're all alone with it, and often can't get the relief they need.

I hope that pain-management courses in medical school will help solve that issue.

Father Robert Kennedy, D.D., Ph.D.

ॐ

Father Kennedy is chair of the theology department and instructor in Japanese language at St. Peter's College in Jersey City, New Jersey. A Jesuit priest, he also practices clinical psychology in Manhattan and in Connecticut. I interview him at his brother's home in West Florida.

How is it that you came to teach Japanese?

I lived in Japan for eight years as a young man. I did some studies there, and discovered Zen Buddhism. I worked with a Japanese teacher in Kamakara, and ten years ago I was installed by the Buddhists as a Japanese teacher, even though I was not a Buddhist. That was something of a first, and it shows the greatness of their generosity in reaching out—to make someone who is not even a Buddhist one of their teachers, a person who will then decide who will teach Buddhism in the future. So I have very close ties with the Buddhists, and my main work, as I see it, is interfaith work in the Buddhist-Christian Community, as well as other interfaith work. Last year I went with a group of students to Auschwitz, reaching out to develop interfaith work in the Jewish-Christian community.

What can you tell me about the similarities and differences between Buddhist and Christian views of suffering?

Well, suffering in the Buddhist tradition is important because the first noble truth of Buddhism is the recognition that all things suffer. Buddhists say that we suffer because we are coming apart. Compartmentalizing. There is no principle of unity. Everything separates and dies. The start of Buddhism is this sensitivity to suffering and the desire to alleviate it where possible. Not everyone has this sensitivity; therefore Buddhists do not expect that all people will be Buddhists. It's a compassionate outreach to the other precisely as other, not because they're a relative or friend, but as other. I often think of this recognition of the other in the terms of the Jewish philosopher Emmanuel Levinas. Humanity begins when we see suffering in the face of the other, and, then, in response to that suffering, we become the Messiah. The Messiah is not someone who comes in the future, but who is present in us when we are responsive to suffering in the face of the other. So back to Buddhism. This sensitivity to suffering is foundational and Buddhism is quite modern in this. Of course, I can't speak for the whole of Buddhism, but this is my understanding of it.

Now, it's fairly traditional to say that we do not know the meaning of things, and, therefore, we don't know the meaning of suffering any more than we know the meaning of happiness. In that world of nondetermination that physics presents us with, each moment is quite unique. Each moment is quite undetermined, and we cannot say why suffering arises. We cannot say what meaning it has, either globally or in the life of an individual. It's entirely relative and transient. We want to give it a meaning. We want to be sure, certain, of things. We like to know the reason for things. Of course, this shows up in the Book of Job, the greatest of the Israeli poets. Why do the innocent suffer? And there is no answer. God does not give an answer. The same question was asked at Auschwitz. Why did these innocent people meet such a fate? There is no answer, finally, to it. Certainly

Buddhism would say that there is no answer. We are just confronted with the fact, moment by moment, that there is suffering.

You talked about things "coming apart." Do you mean by that "entropy"—the tendency of things toward maximum disorder—the opposite of the Taoist and quantum views in which something, some force, runs through everything and ties it together?

The three marks of Buddhism are suffering, impermanence, and soullessness, and of course these are connected. We suffer because we are impermanent, and we are impermanent because we have no soul, no center. But on a deeper level than that there is the Buddhist teaching of emptiness, that the point is not that things will dissolve, but that fundamentally there are no things. That in this moment-by-moment existence, as the universe springs forth each moment is unique, and basically we have energy and light, but we certainly have no "thing." This, of course, has to be taken into consideration when we think of suffering and lack of meaning in suffering. How can there be meaning in suffering in a world in which, really, fundamentally, there is no causality?

And yet it seems we have come to make certain assumptions about pain and suffering—in particular, the assumption that it is redemptive, that it purifies, that it prepares the soul, that it is part of a definite plan. In some quarters, a certain amount of pain and suffering is thought to be a good thing, to strengthen you. This is reflected in the popular phrase "If it doesn't kill me, it makes me stronger." In the war on pain, there does seem to be set of folks who have the attitude that maybe it should not be completely relieved. Maybe it shouldn't be relieved at all.

Sometimes we find that we do not regret having suffered. We may regret the suffering as we go through it, but we realize that having suffered we have become far more human. How could we understand suffering in another if we had not had some suffering ourselves? It is hard to imagine a person who has *no* sensitivity to suffering, who has never suffered. Such a person might be very shallow, you know. Imagine saying, "This is my wife, who has no understanding of suffering." (*laughing*) There is a point where we do not regret having suffered because it has had some good effects in us. This is not to say that it cannot also be completely destructive. How it is handled is important.

I was deeply touched by the writings of Ettie Hillesum, the Jewish woman who died in Auschwitz and whose memoirs were published as *An Interrupted Life*. She grapples with suffering and refuses to be broken by it. In an absolutely extraordinary diary she says she wishes to be the "thinking heart" of the barracks, and that she will not be turned into someone who hates. She says she knows that those who hate have good reason for doing so, but she asks, "Why must we always take the easiest way?" She refuses to hate. She remains compassionate to the suffering around her and doesn't focus exclusively on her own suffering, terrible though it was. So there is a mystery there. Some suffering can be helpful to us. And it is almost inevitable. The development of the human spirit in matter, the refinement of the human spirit—how could it possibly be done without some effort and pain as we mature and grow? So I think all traditions recognize a redemptive quality in suffering.

When you say mature and grow, I can't help thinking about change. If you watch a tree growing from a seedling to a sapling, as it extends upward, pieces fall off, bark is shed, parts thicken and can no longer be contained. When people grow, they may grow through painful change, through events such as accidents or illnesses, some of which they would rather have avoided, but without which they would surely not be the kind of human being they are. Yet it seems that in health care there may be a failure to distinguish between the pain of an upward, positive growth, and the pain of degradation and the downhill spiral of life. The latter demands the kind of compassion that makes us human, but that compassion may be hard to find, either as a result of the system, or the people in it.

You mention the breaking out that change requires. We tend to live in a very small world. I was thinking of the wonderful exchange between God and David in the Jewish scriptures. David decides he's going to build a house for God. The Jewish writers put into the mouth of God the wonderful phrase *"You* are going to build a house for *me?"* When we recognize our smallness, the pain can be terrible. We can lose our moorings when our understanding of God tumbles from the niche where we have put it. This can be frightening. This fear can lead people to a type of fundamentalism where they reassert the truths that they believe they absolutely know. They can get very fanatical about it, very vicious about it. So this is a problem. Accepting change. As we age, for instance, we are not the men that we were some time ago. We shouldn't be.

Whatever the ultimate meaning of suffering, we should try to alleviate it. In the Christian tradition we are saved; we become ourselves, by the corporal works of mercy, not by a lot of fancy ideas in our head, or by loving God in Heaven, but by feeding the hungry and giving drink to the thirsty and clothing the naked. Finally, that has to be our business. To try and alleviate suffering. Not to say it's good for the person, or that they're going to learn from it, but to do our best to feed and clothe and relieve physical and psychic pain where possible. That's how I see my own work as a therapist, to try and help a person understand what has happened to them, to come to terms with it, to accept it, to make changes that have to be made in their circumstances. As Freud says, to make life a little bit easier.

We do what we can to try and alleviate pain. As teachers, we try to alleviate the suffering of ignorance by giving people a skill, a livelihood, or by helping them to read and have a wider vision of life. Education is one of the greatest possible social works. The hospitals that the Catholic community runs try to alleviate physical suffering in the same way. So we are in the business of alleviating pain, not just telling people it's good for them. We are aware that pain can crush people.

You mentioned the pain of realizing our smallness. In the Taoist tradition, and I believe in the Jewish mystical tradition as well, there is no shame or pain in being a cog in a machine. In fact, there can be solace, satisfaction, and maybe even joy in that. Does that make sense?
Yes.

You also mention that alleviating suffering is the thing even in the face of not knowing why we suffer. Yet in our health care system, in our social conscience, maybe even in our cultural mores, we have lost sight of the simple nuts-and-bolts business of alleviating suffering. That clarity of vision has been clouded by issues of finance, organization, allegiance, professional status, politics.

In the Catholic world, and of course outside it, there is the hospice movement, where we simply help people die comfortably and with dignity, and without useless extraordinary medical techniques. This is what Mother Teresa was trying to do in India. There was no thought of curing her people. She was about cleaning them up and loving them and helping them to die in peace. She's been criticized by some for that, but given the resources she had, there wasn't much more that she could do than cut through the bureaucracy and find a way for them to die with dignity.

In the deepest sense, nurturing and loving someone is the highest, best you can do. A physician might argue for medication, but medical care and loving kindness should not, must not, be put in apposition. The medication end of things is being done reasonably well, at least in this country, but the other seems lacking.

That brings us back to the Buddhist notion of sensitivity. There are wonderful personalities who have other gifts, but sensitivity may not be among them. I was reading the other day about Churchill. Despite his wonderful ability to lead a nation, he was not, as Franklin Delano Roosevelt's biographers recount, sensitive to people's feelings. We can't criticize people for not having this kind of sensitivity, but usually those who do gravitate toward helping people. Sometimes all we can do is put our arms around people and hold them and let them know they have a friend. This doesn't, as you say, preclude the other work. Hospitals and the care they provide are critically important. Yet at the end, we all die, and we all need someone just to be with us, touch us, remind us who we are.

Do any examples from your practice come to mind?

I came to therapy rather late in life, a second degree after theology. I was deeply touched by the training I received in clinical psychology. What we had to do was learn how to listen. It was not a question of teaching people things, not a question of telling them what was wrong with their lives, but rather of learning to listen exquisitely to where they were coming from. If we did this well enough, they would eventually tell us what was wrong with them. I think the whole therapeutic method started by Freud is wonderful. Not to pass judgment, just to listen deeply.

Firenze, one of Freud's disciples, had this tremendous sensitivity to people, and was willing to listen, and to learn to listen. We can trust people that they can take care of themselves, that they know themselves. We mustn't override what they think about themselves and tell them what they should think, or what they should feel or what they should believe. I'm very grateful to the clinicians who helped me in my training.

And yet, somehow, these days it can happen that a person, a patient, may be deprived of the right to modulate or moderate or control the way they feel, and be forced to abdicate that responsibility, that power, to someone else. To my eye it is a strange contract into which we have entered with our health care professionals. We accept the notion that they—our therapists, our nurses and doctors—know better than we do what is good for us. The notion that someone else should have control over our own suffering flies in the face of a lot of spiritual beliefs.

This is something that I've thought about and taught about. Patients in pain, elderly people, often try and please the doctor. They are afraid that if they go against the doctor's wishes the doctor will be less available to them and therefore they abdicate more than perhaps they should and go along with what the doctor wants. Those who care for patients have to be careful that the freedom, the independence and the judgment of the patient are constantly respected. I teach some of my students, many of whom are the first generation in their family to go to college, that they have the obligation to stand up for an aged parent or grandparent in the health care setting, particularly when there is any question of experimentation. It's critical that patients *understand* all that is involved. Do they know the difference between therapeutic and nontherapeutic intervention? Do they have complete freedom to back out anytime they wish without fear of annoying a doctor or his staff? Many doctors do wonderful work, but may have no ethical training or background. We cannot, therefore, presume that their decisions are always the ones we would like to have them make for us or for our loved ones.

I guess in the end it all boils down to people being kind to others.
Finally, it comes down to being a mensch.

John Sarno, M.D.

❧

Dr. John Sarno is Professor of Clinical Rehabilitation Medicine at New York University School of Medicine. He is also the author of three best-selling books on back pain and other psychosomatic illnesses. I interview him at his apartment in New York City.

Tell me what you make of the recent reported increase in chronic pain in the United States.

It is not so terribly recent. It has probably been going on for about thirty-five years. If you go back to the fifties and early sixties, there was no such thing as chronic pain, except among people who were dying of cancer and things of that sort. The population of chronic pain sufferers today are people who have pain in the back, the neck, the shoulders, the arms or legs, that is attributed to a large variety of structural abnormalities. I became interested in this subject in the mid-1960s, when I took over as head of the outpatient service at the Rusk Institute of Rehabilitation Medicine. I saw quite a few people in pain, and while physiatrists traditionally treat pain with nonsurgical methods, I was thoroughly disappointed with the results I got using conventional treatment for conventional diagnoses.

I resolved to take a closer look, to doubt the diagnoses, and when I did, I realized that in classic back and neck complaints, we seemed to be dealing with a muscle problem. When I first started to write about this for the literature, I referred to the emotional, psychological, and muscle components by calling it tension myositis syndrome. In my first book on the subject, which came out in 1984, I described the physical disorder, and I briefly described the personality types that seemed to be prone to it, but I really couldn't pin it down. I realized that the problem encompassed more than the muscles in the back, that it also involved nerve tissue, which is why so many people with back pain also had sciatica and why so many people with neck and shoulder pain also had pain in the arm and hand. I saw that a large number of tendon problems that had been attributed to overwork and overuse—of course I'm not talking about a major league pitcher here, just someone who plays tennis on weekends—were involved as well.

It became clear that these complaints were psychologically induced, and that they were the result of something going on in the unconscious. In the book that I published in 1991, I said that this pain is actually produced in the brain as a response to something in the unconscious. By the time I wrote the third book, the one that came out in 1998, I concluded that we were dealing with manifestations of rage in the unconscious mind. This rage seems to be primarily the result of pressures people put on themselves, either to be perfect—with all the ramifications of that, conscientious, hardworking, responsible, achieving, successful—and/or to be good, with all the ramifications of that—a nice guy, a good guy, a helpful person, and so on. These have turned out to be the primary psychodynamics involved. The question is why they lead to pain.

The answer is that there is in each and every one of us a leftover child primitive. From a social and political point of view, what you are seeing here is the result of the continuing influence of that child primitive on human behavior. From a medical point of view, what we are seeing is a conflict between that part of us which Freud called the superego—ethical, moral, intellectual, rational—and the irrational side of us that doesn't want to be perfect and good, the side that doesn't care about any of that stuff—the greedy, self-centered side that wants to be taken care of and indulged. My personal view is that the problems that we are facing in the world right now are the result of the overindulgence of this latter side, an obsession with success and money, ignoring the poverty and suffering in the world. We're supposed to be a Judeo-Christian society, but we don't pay any attention to Judeo-Christian precepts any more.

Medically, chronic pain is waxing because psychosomatic illnesses will increase in grand fashion if they are in vogue, if they have been misdiagnosed by the medical profession, and if treatment for them will be paid for. A clear example is the epidemic of whiplash in Norway, which has one of the most generous and lenient medical insurance programs in the world. Call it whiplash, and the treatment is paid for. All of a sudden, everyone is suffering whiplash. Look at countries where the treatment for whiplash isn't paid for, and there is no incidence of whiplash at all. When this point was made in Norway, there was an outcry among patients who denied that they were faking. The point is that they were not faking. They were suffering from a real syndrome, a psychosomatic illness which was misdiagnosed and unrecognized and therefore allowed to spread in epidemic fashion. Same thing with fibromyalgia, which has, as of this date, involved six million Americans, mostly women. In 1980, it didn't exist. Twenty-one years and we have an epidemic! Why? Because it is psychosomatic and doctors have no idea.

Are you saying that the diagnosis of fibromyalgia didn't exist before 1980, or that the symptoms didn't exist?

The term. Right now I'm working on a book about the psychological dimensions of psychosomatic illness, and, as background, I have re-read all of Freud. Freud described what I call tension myositis syndrome (TMS) back in 1895. The problem was that instead of recognizing that the brain initiated the physical process—which I have done—he said that symptoms were organic and that the psyche was using them to further its own neurotic interests. Fibromyalgia is nothing more than a severe form of TMS. Carpal tunnel syndrome (CTS)? Same thing. Sporadic cases until the mid–80s, when people began to get it and blame it on working on a computer. Nobody in medicine ever asked why the millions of men and women who pounded typewriters since the turn of the century never developed CTS.

In the late 1980s I got a call from a patient of mine, an employee rather high up at the *New York Times*. He told me that they were seeing a lot of CTS and he wondered whether it might not be related to my work. I asked him to send me information on the claims, and he did, and oh my God, it was so classic! These were the same kind of people who got the back pain and the neck pain and the shoulder pain and so on. I called him and told him that it was very likely that it was another psychosomatic manifestation, and I offered to see some of these people without charge, for the purposes of establishing if this was in fact what was going on. Do you know what happened? Nothing! The people wouldn't come to see me. They didn't want to hear of it. So all this is really quite incredible. It's bad enough that the doctors don't know what they're looking at, but the poor patients will not accept the idea either.

They were too interested in manifesting rage to stop?

That's not the way it works. The rage is unconscious. The physical symptoms—and pain is only one, albeit perhaps the most important now, but others may be headache and gastrointestinal problems—are a strategy designed by the brain to prevent the rage from coming to consciousness. All unconscious emotions, particularly those that are unacceptable, are kept repressed. Paradoxically, the psyche thinks it is doing the individual a favor, because it sees pain and these other symptoms as preferable to ruining his life with unbridled rage. Keep in mind it is rage we're talking about here, not anger. Rage! And it is universal, which is why everyone has something that is psychosomatic. It is anger generated inside because one part of oneself, this inner child, cannot bear being put under pressure. This is my theory. You won't find it in the psychiatric or psychological literature, but the authors of such work haven't seen 11,000 patients over the last twenty-eight years. I have. Psychiatrists and psychologists, who like to think that they know something about psychosomatic medicine, don't really know because patients suffering these disorders don't go to them; they go to family doctors, orthopedists, and physiatrists.

Do you see that as a crisis of medical education?

Let me start by saying that in the first half of the last century there seemed to be some awareness of the importance of psychological factors in health and illness. The champion of the notion was Franz Alexander, the founder of the Chicago Institute of Psychoanalysis.

A student of Freud.

Yes, but when you read his writings you see he moved far beyond Freud. In essence, he said that psychological factors were responsible for hyperthyroidism, hypertension, migraine headache, a whole bunch of things.

Then came the Descartian split of mind and body.

That always existed, but around mid-century, medicine became increasingly laboratory-oriented. That was fine, but it seems as though there was an almost total reversal in medicine's interest in psychosomatic matters. For example, it is now believed that ulcers are due to bacteria. Ulcers are still psychosomatically induced.

You're saying the bacteria has only an opportunistic role?
Yes.

You seem to be suggesting a new slant on the usefulness of pain, one that transcends the traditional notion that pain is useful as a warning knell. In what way is it adaptive for the mind to employ pain as a means of avoiding other, more dangerous, emotions?
I see what you're saying. That's very very good. But it's an opportunistic thing. I don't think the brain decides oh, pain is useful. I think the brain realizes that it could serve this purpose, and that it has been allowed to do it in epidemic proportions. We must use the word epidemic.

Everything else you've said is clear, but I'm confused about that last point. The notion of the brain opportunistically employing a tactic makes me think that there might be a certain amount of pressure building, and a search for the easiest release, a path of psychic path of least resistance. Why pain? Is it adaptively better than expressing rage?
Yes. The brain thinks it's safer than exploded rage. Remember that Freud described TMS in 1895, and it had been going on long before that. It may be that the media actually helped spread this epidemic.

So it's a manifestation of the information age?
Yes, that's very good. Jared Diamond, the biologist and writer, has said that of all the scientists in the last two hundred years, only two, Darwin and Freud, synthesized things in a way that was absolutely indispensible. Both those giants used their eyes

and ears to come up with new notions. It was their observational and synthetic brilliance that did it. Everyone else did work that someone else might have done. Until Freud's time, the best minds in the world had no idea that we had an unconscious. Do you realize that? Hundreds of years? Brilliant!

The idea of the unconscious existed in Plato's time.

But as a philosophical notion, not one expressed in science and medicine. Alfred Adler, who was with Freud for about ten years, comes closest to having seen what I have seen. I am in the tradition of Charcot, Breuer, Freud, Adler, and Alexander. I know that sounds full, but the fact is psychosomatic medicine has been dead. This is a medical tragedy, and I'm trying to bring it back. I'm not going to have any success.

Because it violates the current paradigm.

Of course. Think about the financial ramifications. Think about the pain clinics, the whole kit and caboodle. When I first started to do this work in the early 1970s, you could admit patients and keep them in hospital for a number of weeks, and we got to spend time with tough cases. I remember one woman who had been on a narcotic by hypo for months for her pain. She was open to the idea of pyschosomatic illness. We worked with her daily, in an intensive way, and within seven or eight weeks, the pain was gone. She stopped her drug cold turkey and no withdrawal whatsoever. I saw that and I said to myself oh, now I understand! Withdrawal reactions are psychosomatic reactions to deprivation in people who have become addicted. Pain patients are not addicted.

You mentioned pain clinics. Surely there are people who are in real need who require those clinics and their therapies.

Of course, and people who have real pain should never be deprived of medication. That's just the misconception of people in the medical profession who don't understand what addiction really is. But let me tell you something, my friend. All those folks there for the "neck thing," the "back thing," all those poor people who have had half a dozen operations, they are suffering psychosomatic illnesses.

They are in pain and need relief. The point is not that there is no organic basis for this pain, but rather that the brain can induce organic manifestations at many levels. PMS may be the most benign, for example, but I believe that the brain has a role in inducing all the autoimmune diseases. Of course, there is not a direct causal relationship. It's much more complicated than it is with TMS. In rheumatoid arthritis, for example, a noxious substance is produced that destroys the cartilage. The same thing applies to cancer, and to cardiovascular disease, which are manifest over a longer period of time.

So the medical establishment has created an entire phenomenology around psychosomatic pain and has missed the boat completely.

Completely.

Joseph J. Fins, M.D.

ℭℴ

Dr. Joseph Fins is Director of Medical Ethics, and Chief of the Division of Medical Ethics at New York Presbyterian Hospital–Weill Cornell Medical Center. I interview him at his office at the hospital.

Ameliorating a patient's suffering lies at the heart of what a physician is supposed to do, and therefore must be of great interest to a medical ethicist.
You know, there's a painting by Picasso. I believe it's called "Science and Charity," which shows a patient on his deathbed with a nun on one side and a doctor on the other. That synthesis of caring and curing is just what we would like to see in medical practice. Unfortunately, with all the tremendous excitement about the new technologies, we've gotten to the point where we embrace a sort of immortality, a sense that there's no disease we can't cure. This balance of curing and caring that the painting shows has been distorted. Now it's all about trying to cure. The old saying "No pain, no gain," is emblematic of that. You would think such a balance would be a central mandate of medical practice and physician responsibility, but unfortunately it's not.

Too often we don't see pain as the medical emergency that it is. There are a lot of politics involved, and there are concerns about addiction. The war on drugs is often confused with the war on cancer pain. You can see that with the recent concern over the diversion of certain opioids. I don't think it's fair that patients who

222

are dying of cancer, or people who have chronic pain, should be further victimized by repressive law-enforcement tactics that deprive them of beneficial medications. The scourge of drug addiction has had an impact on how we look at pain management and also physician responsibility.

I do not believe that the DEA thinks they interfere with physicians treating patients.

As in many things, perception is important. I know it's not exactly what we're talking about, but the recent activities of the Office of the Inspector General regarding the length of stay in hospice led to a decrease in the referral rates to hospice, and the length of time people were actually there. So, perceptions often have an impact on behavior. The Pain Relief Promotion Act, which was recently before Congress, would have had the DEA going into hospitals looking at how opioids were being used to make sure they weren't being used for the promotion of physician-assisted suicide. The act didn't pass, but the fact that it came about at all is reflective of this sense that when we use pain medicines we're doing something wrong. Had the act passed, it would have had a huge impact on pain management and the perceptions of doctors.

We spent the last twenty years telling doctors it was okay to use pain medicine in the treatment of pain, and that if someone was in the process of dying, and their death was hastened by the treatment of their pain, then so be it. That is not physician-assisted suicide. That is not euthanasia. Chief Justice Rehnquist himself, in *Quill v. Vacco*, a case from New York, said that the intention in these cases is the treatment of pain, not euthanasia—that death is a secondary effect. So perception really is important. Whether the DEA intends this or not, physician behavior can be affected by perceptions.

Let's go back to the Picasso painting. The image of a nun on one side of the dying patient and a physician on the other suggests that, at least to Picasso, there was a clear distinction between competence and compassion. My perhaps idealized notion of a physician is of a practitioner who melds the two. No use to the patient if his degree of medical competence isn't high, and no use either if compassion isn't driving him to work in the best interest of the patient.

We see this in psychiatry, where patients who get psychopharmacology—with one of the new, exciting drugs, SSRIs and the like—together with psychotherapy. I would say it's the same with pain management. The patient's psyche, their family's needs, anticipatory bereavement, whatever the issue is, along with competent knowledge of the pharmacology of the opioids or other adjuvant therapy, are synergistic. Unfortunately, just being a nice guy doesn't make you a pain-management expert.

Nor does being a pain-management expert make you. . .
(*laughing*) A mensch.

There are studies that compassionate care increases the effectiveness of pharmacologic and procedural care. That makes sense. Yet somehow we've gotten off the track in bringing the two together.

I disagree. We've made tremendous progress educating doctors. There's a lot more that we need to do, but when I was in medical school there was nothing on palliative care. Now, at Cornell, it's part of the curriculum. We did a project here in New York State where we visited all fourteen medical schools here in the state to assess what they were doing in palliative-care education, and progress *is* being made. Still, there are a lot of challenges. If you think about palliative-care education, it rightly belongs in psychiatry, it rightly belongs in oncology, it rightly belongs in pathology, it rightly belongs in all the clerkships in the third year, and in electives.

In every specialty.

In every specialty. It's everywhere, and it's also nowhere. So the question is where do you put it? It's kind of like professionalism as a medical school topic. It's everywhere, but it's nowhere. We've been struggling with that as medical educators over the last five or ten years—trying to figure out how to integrate it in the curriculum in a way that's meaningful, that gives it substantive time, but doesn't ghetto-ize it into a little course in the first year that is forgotten downstream. There has been a lot of progress, but attitudes are still a major issue. Pain management is not perceived as having the same import as some other things. The patient in pain is not perceived the same way as is a patient with a fever. Medical students will run off and get their blood cultures and do a fever workup, but they don't do a pain workup. A lot of physicians, medical school graduates, know how to treat infections. They may give a round of antibiotics, maybe two rounds, and then call in the infectious disease specialist, but when it comes to pain, they don't have that same level of competence. That's not because opioid management is more *complicated* than antibiotics, it's not. Antibiotics are a lot more complicated. Opioids are all basically similar. They have different modes of onset and strength and so on, but they are essentially the same class of drug. The reason is that we harbor a concern that we're doing something *wrong* when we're treating pain. We're crossing a moral threshold.

That is something that needs to be addressed before we can get to the technical dimensions. We have to win the hearts of medical students and young doctors before we can have a crack at their minds. We have to demonstrate to them that there really isn't anything more gratifying than taking pain from someone in distress. Once you cross that threshold as a physician and you see the relief, the smile on the patient's face, the unburdening, the great sigh of relief from a family member standing in the doorway of a patient's room, after you've seen that, you'll see that really, that was what you were trained to do. That was what you were meant to achieve. Once we've done that, you've won them over. You've converted them to this other realm where curing and caring truly have parity.

Clearly if we had a choice between curing and caring in our own lives, we'd take a cure even if it meant a little pain. But in these situations, we may be talking about people who cannot be cured. We may have to shift our goals of care and make sure that they are caring. Again, curing and caring shouldn't be mutually exclusive; they should be additive.

I would like to think that physicians choose their professions because they care.

Many physicians choose the career because it's a helping profession that brings solace and relief. But other physicians are motivated by wanting to know the "why" of things—why did this person get sick, why did this happen, what is going on, why does this opioid work differently than that one, so why did this person respond differently than that one? Many of us have a scientific curiosity that is coupled with a compassionate urge. That gets back to the need for both compassion and competence together. They work well together. "Compassion" comes from the Latin.

"Suffering with."

"Suffering with." So, you kind of have to be with the patient to understand at some level what is going on. You need to engage. There is no diagnosis without engagement.

Say a guy comes into the emergency room with his bone sticking out of his leg. You needn't have had a compound fracture yourself to see that his leg is busted, figure what it must feel like, and know what to do.

What if you're a white physician and it's a black patient? The literature suggests that African-American males going in with broken legs don't get the same kind of pain relief as non-African Americans.

That's an awful thing.
An awful thing. And maybe it happens because there is a little less compassion, a little less "suffering with." I don't need to break my leg to know that it probably hurts. But I do need to understand the social context of people coming in, and issues of racial disparities in health care and how that might play out. So it's more metaphorical perhaps than actual.

Isn't it true that most doctors get involved in a cohort after medical school from whom they learn how to behave?
The most important determinant of how people behave and the kind of practice that they engage in is not the influence of the professional societies that many people join, but rather role models in medical school and residency. There's good literature on this, and it's why certain foundations, when they were investing in the end-of-life care movement, invested in the creation of young-to-middle career physicians who could be role models for improved pain-management and palliative care.

What you said earlier about fever and pain is interesting, as pain doesn't generally seem to be regarded as a life-threatening entity or as a disease.
We know that patients in the hospital with untreated pain may have a shorter life expectancy.

And yet there does seem to be a distinction drawn between pain and an organic disease process visible on a test or a scan.
It's a good point. There are two things to consider. One is that the Joint Commission, the body that accredits all hospitals, has just this year established pain as a fifth vital sign. That means that any hospital that wants accreditation, which means basically

all hospitals, is now going to have to assess pain. That's a huge step forward. It's an external force saying that pain is something that needs to be measured. There is, of course, the issue of measurement. There is a visual analog scale. The problem is, let's say you really let your emotions out, you wear them on your sleeve, and you say you have nine out of ten pain [on that scale], the doctor might think, well, I'm going to treat this person as if his pain were a five. Conversely, a stoic John Wayne type who won't admit that his pain is killing him might say his pain is a two. The doctor might treat it as a ten.

This leads to the distinction between pain and suffering. Pain is that physical thing. Suffering is what it means to you, how much it threatens your ego, your "I." I'll give you an example. Say you have really bad neuropathic pain from a toothache. You would rate it as a nine out of ten. You go to the dentist's office Monday morning after suffering with it all weekend, and you're just praying that dentist will be in the office. The nurse tells you that the doctor had a cancelation and can see you in half an hour. Right away, you're not likely to say the pain is at a nine out of ten anymore, because that threat to yourself is diminished.

How about the professional football player who has a shoulder injury during a game in which he won and a game in which he lost. If he won the game, that shoulder injury is in the service of the championship. If he lost the game, it's "My God, I've got six months of pain, surgery and rehab ahead." It's the exact same physiologic component, but it has taken on a different kind of meaning.

Depending upon whom you ask, we have either a romance with stoicism or a nation of whiners. To what extent do you think external factors overlay the perception of pain, given the fact that we live in a melting-pot country full of subcultures with varying degrees of expressiveness?

All of our reactions are going to be mediated by what's going on out there. From the standpoint of the practitioner, it's important to have a sense of what is normative—to understand where a patient is coming from. You can overread or underread a patient's pain, but you don't want to engage in stereotyping.

That's a tough balancing act.
Very tough.

I understand that developing an addiction to opioid analgesics is rare when patients are properly managed and have no history of addiction. Why are some doctors still hesitant to prescribe them?
Let me give you a reason for that. You talk about the cultural determinants that we have out there. A major one of those is that in our society, we seek to control everything: the timing and manner of our death with the assisted suicide movement, our very mortality by cloning Dolly the sheep, and so on. Now what is the antithesis of control? It's addiction.

So if addiction is the antithesis of control, and doctors live in this Baconian world - to sort of control nature - then to do anything that might somehow lead to a lack of control is really antithetical to what we're all about. This fear of letting go, of being out of control, has a big impact on why we are sometimes hesitant to use these medications.

Robert Jarvik, M.D.

०१०

Dr. Robert Jarvik is the president of Jarvik Heart Inc., a pioneer in the field of artificial heart technology. I interview him at his corporate office in New York City.

You're in the artificial heart business. The heart is the metaphorical seat of feeling. What have you learned about doctors and chronic pain?

People have a lot of social baggage about pain. For some doctors, managing it is primary, for others it's very secondary. Some doctors would like to help out of pure compassion, some would like to but feel that they can't for various reasons, some consider it to be a nuisance and don't particularly care whether the patient feels it, and some are going to look at it as a potential addiction problem. My guess is that if you don't worry about the incurable tumor that's causing the pain and you don't worry about addiction but view pain as an incurable condition, if you say, "Look, here's something you can't cure, you can only make it ease off for the time you're treating it," then you can make life liveable and comfortable. So long as you keep in mind the respiratory status and the operation of heavy machinery—areas where the drug might hurt a patient—and so long as the patient understands that there is a degree of compromise, great benefit can be had from using the right medications.

You can't cure the thing that leads a person to need an artificial heart, but you can prolong life with the machine you make. It seems that the difference between managing and curing is important.

Accepting that difference makes things a whole lot better. We have patients who are awaiting a heart transplant. They are what we call "bridge" artificial heart patients. We also have patients who are permanently on the artificial heart. Their attitudes can be very, very different. A person who is waiting for a transplant is generically nervous, waiting for the donor heart, wanting the heart that represents the chance to be better. A patient who is permanently on an artificial heart accomodates to that—not only because of their physical condition but, to quite an extent, because of their personality—and in certain ways they have a better circumstance. The longest artificial heart patient was offered a transplant and turned it down. He has a totally wonderful attitude toward life and accepts all of the issues of it. He is mobile, he lives at home, he has a relatively normal life except that he lives with the inconvenience of carrying and charging batteries that weigh a couple of pounds. But he is very strongly influenced by attitude. I remember a couple of earlier bridge-transplant patients, one of whom had a wonderful life, he lived about eleven years after the transplant. He went back to work, he went dancing with his wife all the time, he lived a good life on that donor heart. But another guy, who was transplanted about the same time, lived in constant fear that the heart would reject. He was just really unhappy, and he didn't survive more than a year or two. He was very unhappy in pretty much the same circumstance.

The patient's attitude toward pain not only affects how the patient deals with their pain, but how the outside world responds to them as well. If one accepts something with finality, namely that this type of pain comes from an incurable condition, that it's going to be medication forever, then, if you have that attitude, I don't see why it should be a problem. Then it just comes down to the choice of procedures or medications, which have the least side-effects, which do the best job while doing the least harm.

So acceptance, which is a part of the grieving process, applies both to transplant patients and chronic pain patients?

Let me give you another nice analogy from the heart situation. The patient who has lived the longest on our latest heart, the Jarvik 2000, is a clinical psychologist. He ran a program in palliative care for AIDS and cancer patients. He was with something like 150 patients at the moment of their death. His experience of seeing his own body fall apart, of expecting death with such certainty before the artificial heart became an option really shows a lot. Once he reached the point where he accepted that he was going to die very soon, it was very hard for him to go the other direction, to seize an opportunity to do something that would give him a chance to live again. He didn't want to get his hopes up and be disappointed. Reaching the point of accepting death once has really helped him enormously with what he calls his "extra" life. Now, he goes about living without undue concern. Things don't stop him. He knows that there are risks and troubles and he knows he's not totally fine, but he has such a good attitude because he reached the point where he gave up. If pain patients don't seek a cure, but rather understand that the pain is always going to be with them and seek to ease it as much as possible, they're likely to do much better.

When we talk about the issues of getting regulatory approval for an artificial heart, and you talk about what it means to someone who faces certain death without it, even a modest improvement is good. Of course, nobody *wants* merely a modest improvement, they just accept it if it's all there is. But when you can talk about something that's much more than a modest improvement, when you can talk about *real* rehabilitation in a heart disease patient, giving them real exercise tolerance, mobility, all the things that they've lost, plus recovery of some of the function of the heart, then you find that hope comes back, and, with it, attitude improves.

One thing this book might do for people in chronic pain is to bring them examples of people who have given up on a cure for their pain and focused on good treatment for their pain, gotten the right result, come out the other side, had a life after the debilitating phase of chronic pain, started at ground zero and reached a liveable place. That's something that can really help.

Let me ask you a question. Have you ever negotiated with yourself?

Of course. Everybody has.

And with other people?

Naturally.

Then you know that the way you win a negotiation is to be totally willing to lose. As soon as you realize you are negotiating for a point that you can just walk away from, you can be very effective. A person has to really walk away from the pain-free past they've lost, not mourn the past, not complain. Once something has happened to them that's bad enough to give them chronic pain, they have to change their attitude. They have to take the best of what's left in their life, push the pain out, and don't complain about it.

If a pain patient accomplishes this inner change, is there a change in the way others regard them as well?

I think that occurs all the time. People create their own self-fulfilling prophecy. They're treated better if they act better. Although there are people who have the right to demand certain things, acting in a demanding way leads to resistance and dislike. People who are in a fairly dependent circumstance don't do well by being demanding, and they don't do well by being meek and pitiful, either. They do better by being a real up-front person, not playing any of those stereotypes.

Of course, I'm talking here about the relationship between a chronic pain patient and their caregiver, not someone who is in an acute situation. If you've been injured and you're pleading for help, obviously that's a different kind of pain and a different story. I'm talking about long-term accommodation in a person who has the need for chronic medication. Also, let's say they're being treated with a sincere effort, and being given the dose of medication that is the most that can be given, and they keep saying, "It's not enough, it's not enough, I gotta have more," then the interaction with the people who are treating them is going to be bad. If, on the other hand, they say, "I know that's all you can do, I'm getting on okay with it, but I wish we could find something that would do a little better," they're going to be received differently.

On the other hand, if someone realizes there is a procedure or a medication that can help them, but they're too meek to say, "I really have reason to believe that this is going to help and this is why. Why won't you do this, please? It's necessary, I need it, please do it, or tell me where I'm wrong, why it can't possibly work, but just don't let me think that there's something there, not far off, that could really help, but I'm not getting it," then they should get a good result, too. Of course, all this is with the bias of my own personal style, because I believe that directness is best. Not everyone is like that, but if people are up-front with themselves when they have a really devastating situation, they are more likely to be able to get through it and start anew. Every artificial heart patient is at that point, goes through this process, and, of course, we're not just at the place of "live a little longer"; we're at the place of rehabilitation to normal health. The pain patient's frustration is similar. Frustration is a tough one. It eats people alive. When you combine it with pain it's even tougher.

Pain is so experiential, it is hard to communicate.

It's very hard to imagine something you've never felt before. Years and years ago, the department of artificial organs that I worked at had a program going on in artificial vision. They were doing brain stimulation in blind volunteers. They put electrodes on the visual cortex and stimulated it with different wave forms. The patient would be conscious at the time, under local anesthesia. There was a volunteer who wasn't blind, and he had this stimulation done. He could see, but he was willing to undergo this procedure for research purposes. He came to work in the program later, and he said that when he was stimulated, he saw a new color. Absolutely, he had never seen that color before and has never seen it since. It was a new color. I asked him, So, was it like purple, like orange? He couldn't say. But it was vivid and clear, and it was a new color. And it wasn't like it was in the spectrum. Of course, I believed him completely, but it was an experience, because of something that happened in the brain, that another person couldn't readily picture. So people who treat people with pain should recognize that they pretty much don't know what the patient is talking about. They can't, unless they've been there.

Especially in the case of chronic pain, which often lacks the obvious source evident in the acute pain of a burn or an accident.

But the patient, for their own self-esteem, and ability to cope with it, is perfectly justified in saying, "I am the best expert in the world on my own pain. I know what I'm talking about. I know what it feels like. I know what it is. Nobody knows it better." Many of the people they're dealing with have only dealt with such pain secondhand, through description. Physicians can think of the worst pain they can remember, when something really hurt, and say to themselves, "Maybe it's like that." But maybe it isn't. Still, this "expertise" shouldn't make the patient rude and demanding, which some patients can be. You want to get the frustration and anger out somehow. You, the patient, want to remember what it was like to be a decent and reasonable person who was not controlled and distracted by the pain. You want to try and remember how you dealt with people. Even though it's hard to do, you have to at least pretend you're your old self. That may key the responses of others and make them better. You don't want to be dealt with as a "pain patient"; you want to be dealt with as a person.

Madeline Ko-i Bastis, R.N.

ෙ

Madeline Bastis is a Zen Buddhist priest, and the first Buddhist to be board certified as a hospital chaplain. She trained at Memorial Sloan Kettering Cancer Center, New York University Medical Center, and in the AIDS section of the Nassau County Medical Center. She is the founder and director of the Peaceful Dwelling Project, a not-for-profit foundation seeking—through workshops, meditations, and retreats—to improve the quality of living for people with life-challenging illnesses and their caregivers. I interview her on a park bench on Long Island, in summer.

What have you learned about pain from the people who have come to you for help?

Everyone suffers pain. Whether it's physical, spiritual, or emotional, it is our lot to have pain. How we look at pain determines how much we suffer. I've seen people suffer keenly and others with the same affliction manage to hold in their pain. For most people, our first reaction is to contract, to push away the pain, either physical or emotional, because clearly we don't want it. I've learned that there is a way of befriending the pain, of giving the pain space to exist. It is possible to live with pain and accept it.

Do people ever say to you that their pain has a purpose in their life?

Some individuals who have a very strong spiritual practice may find a meaning in pain, but, in general, very few people do. Pain is a dirty word. People don't like to use it. People want to find a way to get rid of pain rather than to give it space. They want to stop it, and they try medications and other things. One of the difficulties for people suffering difficult pain is that they feel they are the only ones, that they're isolated, that they're lepers. So, one of the meditations I do with people who are dying involves thinking of all the other people who are feeling the exact same way they are feeling at that moment and to breathe in their pain, to take it in, and to send out light, bright, cool healing. Many of the people who are willing to do this feel that they are no longer isolated in their pain. They feel connected. They realize that others are feeling the same way they are, and feeling the same pain. So they become a part of a community.

When I was a trainee and first went into a cancer hospital, it scared me to be near people who were suffering a lot because I wanted to do something for them and frequently I couldn't. What you have to do in that case is to just learn how to be with it. But first you have to learn to accept that you have your own fear that some day you are going to feel that way too. I think all of us have that, and that it is one of the reasons why most people try as much as possible to avoid being near people with pain.

Are you saying that people are able to heal themselves through a spiritual practice, or are you talking about temporarily dulling the keen edge of agony?

It has to do with the question you asked before. It has to do with finding a meaning in pain. This particular meditation is called *tonglen*. That means taking and sending. It's like sending your pain to the dry cleaners. You start with your own pain. You see it in front of you as an entity. The image used is hot, heavy, dark smoke. You breathe in hot heavy and dark, and you send out light bright and cool. Many people feel their throat constrict, but they feel the smoke getting lighter. Then I ask them to imagine all the other people feeling the same way, and to breathe in *their* smoke and send it out lighter. They do that for a while, and then I tell them to feel love and acceptance back from all the folks they've helped. It's a very moving experience.

We send what we wear to the dry cleaner, but we don't send our skin. Do you see pain as part of us, or as something that can be shed?

I do not see pain as a part of us. I think people make a mistake when they say, "I am an angry person. I am a person who has great pain. I am a person who is suffering." Pain is like sound. It rises and it subsides. We can't control that. What we can control is how we respond to the pain. When I get hurt, I expect the pain to ebb and flow. It's not a solid knot. If one is willing, one can really look at the quality of the pain and see it change. It may be solid and the same all the time.

Years ago I went on a week-long Zen retreat. At 4:30 in the morning we started sitting cross-legged, and we continued until 9:00 at night. It was difficult. On my second day, I had an abscessed tooth. Although there was a doctor there who was able to get me penicillin, it still ached all the time and took my attention. Late that evening I sat down incorrectly, and pulled a muscle in my groin. The pain was so excruciating that my tooth didn't hurt anymore. What I found was that the mind can only handle one thing at a time.

So although I don't believe that we cause our own pain, I do believe we can cause our own suffering by the way we look at our pain. Pain is not something that we deserve, nor something that we bring on ourselves. Conversely, I don't think we should be expected to overcome it. That's something I find difficult in a hospital setting, and even with family members. I lost my younger sister five years ago. For two or three years, she would get dizzy, have to sit down, have to go to the bathroom frequently. She would be faint. People, including me, got annoyed with her, believing it was something in her head. Three years later, she died of the organic cause of those symptoms. The point is, we tend to think, "Okay, you've been in pain for a while, it's enough, get over it. It's enough for you and it's enough for me, and I don't want to deal with it."

So our intolerance of others' pain has its roots in our discomfort with our own?

I think so. I have a friend who is a well-thought of Buddhist teacher. I respect him very much. Once, when I was going to visit a person who was going to have surgery to remove a tumor in his throat, this teacher told me to tell the cancer patient not to have chemotherapy because it would be painful and unpleasant. My response was "Look; each person has their own path. My job isn't to tell him what to do, but rather to be there and be present for what this person desires." My teacher couldn't see it. He expected this patient to be—and this is his word—"gallant." I hate that word. We have no right to expect anybody to be gallant or Stoic. The most moving moments of my spiritual career have been when I have been with a teacher who was able to shed tears when something happened. To be with a person that way.

As a person who stands at the intersection of health care and spiritual practice, do you think there's a lack of the kind of compassion you have just described in our health care system, our culture, our clergy?

The difficulty is in defining compassion. Many Americans think it means being warm and fuzzy and sympathetic. I prefer the Buddhist definition of compassion, which is "doing the appropriate thing." Clergy have the job of emptying themselves, leaving behind their own preconceptions and prejudices, and doing the appropriate thing. Health care professionals have that job, too, but they're not trained to do it.

When I was becoming a senior Zen student, I was directed to meditate on a koan. The koan was, "How does the great bodhisattva manifest compassion? In the same way as he would reach his hand behind him in the middle of the night to straighten out his pillow." Straightening the pillow is not something you think about; you do it instinctively. For me, as someone who meets with many, many sick, chronically ill, addicted, or dying people, as well as convicts and health care professionals, this is how I see my job. I have to present a clean slate each time I'm with a person. Sometimes it's very hard.

It may be automatic, but for me such straightening evokes the restoration of order. One straightens a pillow because it is crooked or lumped up, because it has drifted away from your back or your head or your knee or wherever you needed it. That koan feels like it might involve putting things back into alignment—fixing something out of kilter.

Oddly enough, I never thought of it that way. I interpret it as a matter of clarity, of just doing what needs doing. For many people that appropriate action is to take medication, by the way. Not everybody can meditate. Now, I'm a recovering alcoholic. When I had a colonoscopy, I made the decision not to take any strong pain medication. I made that decision because I knew my personality. But when I have a headache, I take an aspirin. I don't sit there and feel the pain. If the aspirin doesn't work I sit there and try to handle it, but I never tell people not to take medication.

Recently a woman I've known for several years was dying of cancer. She was in hospice. I drove some distance to see her, because she wanted to do a special meditation for the dying. When I got there I found that they had medicated her to the point where she didn't even recognize me. Now, as a Buddhist, if I am near death, my goal is to be as clear as possible when I die. It's a touchy balance, and one I'd like to be in control of. If I feel I need the pain medication, I can have it, but I'm willing to go to the edge so I can be clear.

Spiritual goals aside, it's a fairly nuts-and-bolts thing you're describing. It's whatever works.

But knowing what will work can be tricky. You want to be like a clear lake in which the right thing bubbles to the surface and recognize it. Instinctive isn't quite right. It doesn't always happen, unfortunately, but when it does, you just know. It's like a sportsman saying, "You're in the zone." You've done your clinical practice and your spiritual practice, but there are those days when the mind is clear and whatever comes up, you're on a roll. It's possible to do something spontaneous with training behind it. A surgeon can be in the zone sometimes, but you have to have clarity, not politics, not any other agenda. But in our health care system, in terms of what I've seen of medical ethics, the primary questions are "Can we be sued?" "Is it cost effective?" "Will we learn anything from this procedure?"

Yet, in all fairness, we cede the responsibility for our care to our caregivers.

We like to think that there is someone who knows more than we do. It's like going to an expert. We expect them to know what to do, and to take everything out of our hands. A lot of us don't want to be in control of pain, treatment, even our lives. We live in a very codependent society.

The irony is that pain is so personal, so individual, and so impossible to share, that the greatest expert on your pain is you.

Ah.

Antonio M. Gotto Jr., M.D.

ℰℐℴ

Dr. Antonio Gotto is Dean of the Weill Medical College and Provost for Medical Affairs at Cornell University. I interview him on a bright autumn day, at his office in New York City.

Has medical education on the management of chronic pain changed in the last ten or fifteen years?

Yes, during the past decade, we have seen some dramatic changes in medical education. We have moved away from emphasizing lectures in favor of smaller discussion groups. Here at Weill Cornell, we refer to this as small group problem-based learning. The aim is to get the medical student not to focus on memorization of facts, but to learn principles and how to apply them, and how to get and analyze information. In addition to that, we have made an effort to emphasize the humanistic aspects of medicine. This is where issues of pain and suffering come into play.

As medicine comes to rely more upon the use of various devices and tests to measure and determine the patient's condition, and less and less upon the patient history, the interview, the physical examination, and observation of the patient, we risk, in a serious way, dehumanizing, de-emphasizing the interpersonal relationship between the physician and the patient, which is at the center of how medicine has been practiced for hundreds of years. We have started a program called the Humanities in Medicine here at Weill Cornell, in which we have brought in people involved with specific types of suffering or different types of pain. Let me give you two examples. One is the play *Wit*, which is about an English professor who is suffering from ovarian cancer. Kathleen Chalfont, the star of the play, brought her group here on two occasions and had readings and open discussions with the students, faculty, and staff about dealing with cancer, about the suffering involved, about the effect on the individual and their circle. We also brought William Styron and his wife here, and he discussed his experience with near-suicidal depression. Depression is associated with a form of pain, and Styron described this pain and the burden that it represented to him. This program brings the notions of pain and suffering and dealing with the patient as an individual to the forefront of the students' attention.

To appreciate pain and suffering, the physician has to be an acute observer. We have a program in this series also with the Frick Collection, in which we bring students to the Frick Museum. They observe a series of paintings and also photographs of patients with different diseases at different stages in their lives, and then at the end of the session they meet with an art historian and a professor from the medical school and they discuss their observations. This is aimed at using art as a way of honing observation. So pain and dealing with pain have become a part of the curriculum, and this emphasis on the humanistic aspects of medicine, I believe, makes our students much more receptive to discussions and an understanding of pain and suffering.

Our less-than-sympathetic attitudes toward pain and suffering derive in part from a long tradition of believing that people in pain have done something bad, and that their suffering is an external punishment of some kind—that dealing with pain and suffering are part of a character-building process. We have the examples of the stiff-upper-lip Englishman and the centuries-old notion of Stoicism which goes all the way back to the Greeks. The notion that it is a sign of weakness or cowardice to give an emotional response commensurate with the pain has been passed down for generations.

By the way, when I think about cultural aspects of pain, I think back to a trip a group of us physicians took to China back in the late 1970s. We visited the Fu Wei Cardiovascular Center in Beijing. While we were there, we saw patients undergoing open-heart surgery where acupuncture was the anesthesia method. It turns out that these patients were put into a program three months before the surgery in which they were introduced to a mind-set that enabled them to deal with what would ordinarily be a very painful and traumatic procedure. They were getting some light dosage of intravenous anxiety medications. But that was all, whereas in this culture, in Western medicine, such a procedure requires very deep anesthesia.

Western medicine has become primarily a technological art, so I can see that a program in what you call the humanistic aspects of medicine might be a good counterweight to all the technological training. Is there some theme, some course, or even some informal format in which those two poles of the practice are brought together, or is the student expected to make that synthesis on his or her own?

There are cases in which they are brought together. There may be a patient encounter or example of a patient suffering from chronic pain and suffering. I don't remember the name of every course in the curriculum, but I don't think we have one specifically entitled "Pain." Yet pain management is part of the training that a medical student does get in presentations, particularly from the neurology department and the anesthesiology department. These are two areas where specific pain-management programs have arisen. Pain has tended to fall between the cracks between medical specialties, but there is a subspecialty, and at our institution it is within the anesthesiology department, that deals specifically with management of pain. So at the point where a neurologist or a cancer patient or some other specialist is doing all that they know how to do and a patient is still in pain, we have a consultation with a specialist in pain management.

I guess I am still looking for that cohering theme.

The theme starts with the applicant selection process here at Cornell. You can fill up the class with students who have straight As and who score very highly on MCATS but never show a spark of human compassion. We look very carefully at our applicants, at what they have done. Many have been out of university for one or more years; some have worked in the Peace Corps, volunteered in communities, done any number of activities that show that they care for people. We emphasize attention to the whole patient. We start our students with patient contact, going out to physician offices within the first month of medical school—very early clinical experience. On their own, our students man a clinic for the homeless on the East Side. One of our students goes over at 4:30 every morning and serves soup to people who sleep on the steps of the Presbyterian Church on Fifth Avenue. Our students are involved with the poor and the underserved. On their own volition, they organized a program called Remedy in which they raised very large amounts of money to purchase books and computers for a hospital in Tanzania—a hospital which provides care for eight million people or so. Over half of our students take an elective abroad, going to very primitive places, villages, and work there. So we do have a student body that represents positive human values, caring and compassion, and I believe that this results in a product, a practicing doctor, who is more likely to exhibit these characteristics.

Speaking of the poor and the underserved, how do you prepare future doctors for the reality of a health care system dominated by financial con-

siderations, a system that doesn't leave much time for the fostering of a compassionate doctor-patient relationship?

This is the whole reason why we try to select and educate students to have a feeling for the patient as an *individual* rather than a composite of different subspecialties of medicine. This requires spending enough time with a patient to get a feeling of what the individual is like as a whole, and how the various aspects of the patient's personality may reflect some underlying disease but also may suggest to the physician a more comprehensive approach rather than carving out and focusing on one organ system. In our electives we emphasize complementary medicine, which means in addition to the traditional forms of medical practice, other adjuncts are used, including counseling, meditation, in some cases acupuncture, in some cases the use of herbals.

Regardless of how a doctor may feel about his or her patient, regardless of how comprehensive and insightful his or her observations, if that doctor is working for an HMO that gives him nine minutes with a patient, care is going to be constrained. Are you fostering a desire to change the current system?

There has been a shift away from capitation, from managed care. The patients have pulled back, the insurers have pulled back, the physicians have pulled back. What the health care gurus were predicting in the late eighties and nineties has never come about. I don't think our graduates would practice very well under that type of system, and I don't think most of them will have to. Now if you are saying that things will be homogenized and this is what everyone will end up with, I would have to say one can practice medicine in many different situations, but this is so alien to the way we train our students that if they are left to any kind of choice, I think they would elect to practice differently.

Patients who complain about their pain, whose pain is not ameliorated or controlled in the first or second round of therapy, are often labeled whiners or drug-seekers and shunted from doctor to doctor. Why do you suppose that happens?

Pain management is very difficult. Musculoskeletal symptoms are among the most common patient complaints, and the most common cause of lost work time. These problems are often very difficult to deal with, particularly when a diagnosis is not immediately obvious. The experience of an illness itself has an effect on the emotions and psyche of a patient, but the emotions and psyche have an effect on the course of an illness as well. There is evidence, for example, that depression can suppress the immune system. There are studies at Duke University and elsewhere that show the effects of faith, prayer in some cases, on patient survival. This is a somewhat controversial area, but there are credible data to show that cancer patients, for example, who have a positive attitude have a better chance of surviving than those who don't. Sometimes in treating cancer there is a very narrow margin between killing the cancer and killing the patient with the treatment. These are difficult concepts to explore in a scientific experiment, but I don't have any doubt myself that the will and spirit of the patient, the psyche, is an important aspect of health and disease and an important component in treatment and recovery.

Some of the pain patients I interviewed for this book made the observation that although they would never wish their pain on anybody, they felt that if their physician could have their back, their liver, or their leg for a day, that physician's practice of pain management, including any fears or prejudices about dependence upon opioid analgesia, would dramatically change.

Those patients make a very good point. I don't think a physician needs to go through every therapy or test that they prescribe for their patients, but it is difficult to have a proper level of understanding or empathy for someone if you've never had any experience with their condition. You see this in families. I have seen this in my own family, with two of my daughters. There are some families that don't seem to have much illness, and when illness suddenly strikes, they have a much more difficult time adapting to it than perhaps some family that has had several experiences with it. I have found that where there is a child who has some serious chronic, painful illness, maybe life-threatening or fatal, there is tremendous stress on the family. It either draws the family closer together or it splits them up. Dealing with chronic illness and chronic pain are synonymous, and are one of the most difficult things that a family unit has to cope with. It is a test of the marriage as to whether it survives it or not.

I wonder whether the same thing couldn't be said of the doctor/patient relationship, which I see as a marriage of a sort. Chronic pain seems to me to stress that relationship too.

It does. The inability to diagnose a chronic illness, the inability to treat the disease and the pain, very much frustrate the physician and the patient both.

And if you add cultural filters, fears of addiction, legal issues, the situation worsens.

There are many barriers to overcome. Treatment of chronic pain is one of the most difficult aspects of medicine. It's difficult from the patient's point of view, from the physician's point of view, and, as you have inferred, it can either disrupt the physician/patient relationship or it can bring doctor and patient closer together.

Patricia M. Good

☙

Patricia Good is Chief of the Liaison and Policy Section of the Office of Diversion Control at the Drug Enforcement Administration— the part of the DEA that deals with licit as opposed to illicit drugs. I conduct the interview at DEA headquarters in Arlington, Virginia.

Why do you think some doctors feel they are scrutinized too carefully by the DEA?

The notion that the DEA somehow monitors the activities of physicians is a myth. There are about eight- or nine-hundred-thousand physicians registered with us, and there are about four-hundred drug-diversion investigators nationwide, out in the field "monitoring" the activities of these nine-hundred-thousand doctors. There is no data system that tracks prescriptions federally, there is no monitoring of the activities of doctors on any level on the DEA's part. We get involved when we are asked to react to a problem brought to our attention by a medical board or by a private citizen, but by and large we do little to no "monitoring" of the physician population.

Why do you suppose people have the perception that there is that scrutiny if it doesn't exist?

There are laws concerning controlled substances and how they have to be handled. While there is an overarching federal law, the Controlled Substances Act, it simply states that controlled substances, when used for medical or scientific purposes, are being used within the scope of the law, but that any use of them outside of that is illegal—is a criminal act. There are also some DEA regulations about the physical handling of the controlled substances, how they have to be stored and tracked in terms of record keeping. At the physician level there is one very simple requirement—that a prescription for them be written by a properly registered person for a legitimate medical purpose. That's the only regulation that applies to a physician.

There is this criminal element that we sometimes investigate—when the activity of a physician is totally outside the scope of legitimate medicine, when they are simply selling drugs as a drug pusher might. There are all kinds of reasons why people do this. For profit, or who knows what. Sometimes it's for sexual favors. So in those instances, yes, we do conduct criminal investigations of doctors who are using their prescribing authority for illegal purposes. We also assist medical boards when they get involved in cases of improper prescribing that result in diversion. In those events we take some administrative action, possibly just write a letter to the doctor and say, "This is a little bit outside the scope; it's causing some problems; your patients are doctor shoppers." It's not a punitive action, but a notice that they should be a little more careful.

There are seventeen states that have passed laws of various types to monitor the prescriptions filled at pharmacies in their state. A few of them did it through the use of paper, triplicate forms, most of them now do it simply by electronic data interchange from the pharmacy to the state agency. There has never been a federal program, and I believe that there are only three states left that even use paper forms. The myth of this onerous thing is largely overstated, and this kind of thing leads to the perception that we monitor everything, because we do see what rises above the surface of normalcy. The state medical boards are more closely involved in monitoring the practice of medicine. That's their main focus in life, whereas it's not ours. Oftentimes people do lump together this body of investigative government people as the DEA, when in fact they're not the DEA. They could be Medicaid fraud investigators. They could be state medical board investigators. They could be who knows who? There are a number of people who investigate the distribution of physician samples. Those folks work for the FDA. They have nothing to do with the DEA, but somehow we get lumped together as the "regulators."

Would you explain the term "doctor shoppers?"

There is big business in selling pharmaceutical drugs on the street. Many of these drugs are highly prized and command large prices. There are rings of individuals who make it their business to go around gaining as many of these drugs as they can from multiple doctors, feigning illnesses, bringing with them doctored-up patient files of real patients. They herd people around the area to get prescriptions cashed in many different pharmacies from many different doctors so they are not easily detected. Their real purpose in life is to sell these drugs illegally.

These people sometimes dupe doctors, because they know how to play the game well. They know what illnesses to feign; they know what symptoms to describe; they know how frequently they can get away with coming back to a doctor. The doctors don't like to find out they've been had by these people. We feel that when we get involved in these cases, we are doing the medical community a service by tracking them down.

Seventeen states have prescription monitoring programs where the data from pharmacies are dumped directly into a state database. Most of those programs are now focusing on patients who are receiving opioids and other prescription, controlled substances from multiple doctors. The programs force these individuals into a treatment plan with one specific physician, so that if there is a real medical issue they get the treatment they need, but preclude them from visiting twenty, thirty, forty doctors, getting outrageous quantities of drugs to sell on the street.

While we see doctor shoppers as people who try to score drugs from multiple doctors, there *are* people who don't get adequate treatment from the first, second, or third doctor they see, and they very likely could go to more than one doctor before they get to the point where they are being treated adequately. We would not presume that these people are getting controlled substances from all the doctors they see, at least not simultaneously.

These people are often termed "pseudoaddicts." Because a person is undertreated, they exhibit drug-seeking behaviors that are usually attributed to the real doctor shoppers or addicts. Until they get adequate treatment, they may exhibit some of these symptoms because they are desperately trying to get the help they need. Many of the prescription-monitoring plans that have monitored this type of behavior have helped the people in the "pseudo" category find adequate help, but get rid of the people out there selling drugs.

Can you help me understand your definition of the term "addict"?
There is a very widespread legitimate use of opioid medications, and the DEA has never had an issue with that proper use. When I use the word "addiction," I'm not talking about the physical dependence that develops in the body when one takes a drug because they need it medically and the body simply adjusts to the dosage. We have heard the medical community define the terms "dependence" and "addiction" very differently. We definitely accept their definitions as being separate and distinct. Anyone who

takes an opioid will become physically dependent, or tolerant, of the substance. That's not to imply that they are addicted or causing some kind of harm or engaging in a socially ill behavior.

When I say "addict," I'm talking about someone who is acting outside the scope of medical treatment, or using the drug for purposes other than pain relief, if we're talking about opioids. They're using them to the point of harm; they have a compulsive need for them. Ever since they were first extracted from the opium poppy, these substances have had a huge following for their euphoric effects. Look back to the Sumerians, look back to the Civil War, and you will see an element of addiction and harm attached to these same products, whether they were initiated as medical treatments or just extracted for their euphoric effects. I've seen lives ruined by drug abuse. I've seen people who never can hold down a job, who cannot have normal relationships with family and friends. Whether it is a pharmaceutical product they are abusing, an opioid, heroin or LSD or some other type of drug altogether, there is a degradation of their quality of life that goes with it. It's a global, societal issue.

Whether it's myth, poor information, or mistaking state agencies for federal agencies, some doctors still do feel an adversarial relationship with the DEA. What other reasons might there be for that feeling?

There are a number of reasons. In years past, medical students were taught to fear the use of opioids for reasons of addiction, and that it was a bad thing to use them, and if they *did* use them, someone would come get them, whether that was the state or the DEA or its predecessor agencies. There was always this overarching notion that someone could get you if you did the wrong thing. What we get lost in is what is the definition of the wrong thing. I've been with the DEA for thirty years, and I when I first started I remember people writing letters saying, "I have a cancer patient and I'm afraid if I give them whatever opioid they'll become addicted. What should I do?" I was stunned that anyone would even ask the question. Why are you worrying about "addiction" when someone has a terminal illness, and why would you think to ask us if it's okay? You're the doctor, you should know. The DEA doesn't regulate medical practice. Never has.

On the other hand there have been some doctors over the years who have gone to jail because their mission in life has been to sell drugs. Case law dating back to the early 1900s clearly says that a doctor acting as a pill pusher can't hide behind their license and expect no ramifications. So every time there is a case where somebody does end up in jail or get sanctioned heavily by a medical board, there's an element of people who wave it in front of everyone and say, "Look. See? They really are out there to get us." Oftentimes they only hear half the story. I don't know of any court or even any prosecutor who would accept a case unless there was overwhelming proof of an illegal activity. We have such a huge presumption of innocence to overcome to ever get to that point—that the person really was just practicing medicine—that to think that we could convict somebody of an illegal drug sale when they're really just practicing medicine is almost ludicrous.

So, unfortunately, the ones that do hit the papers make a big splash and everyone uses them as a rallying cry, and the people who have an agenda to either get regulators off their back, to not have triplicate prescriptions, or to not have prescription monitoring simply wave that around as "Look, they're after us again." We look at our statistical information for a given year, and we arrest fifty out of nine-hundred-thousand doctors, and another fifteen or twenty have their license revoked by unilateral DEA action. That's not really indicative of the fact that we're out there hammering doctors because they made one bad decision. We're looking at people, if we're looking at them, because they have a pattern of dumping drugs onto the street, not because they had one patient that maybe they didn't read right and that person may have been a drug abuser.

Fifty out of nine-hundred-thousand sounds like a tiny percentage, but I would imagine that pain specialists and other doctors who prescribe a lot of opioid medications are a much smaller population than that. Is that right?

Most of the people who are prescribing opioids are general practitioners. It's not limited to pain specialists. In fact, when you look at some of the commercial data that's available on what specialties write prescriptions for opioids, it isn't largely the pain specialists, it's largely non-pain specialists, such as internists, general practitioners, dentists. We saw some data recently that covered every specialty you could imagine, and some you couldn't even imagine being there, like optometrists, who in some states can write prescriptions. So anyone who is registered with us to write Schedule II drugs can write for opioids. It's not limited to certain specialties. Oncologists, surgeons, orthopedic specialists: the list goes on.

Is opioid use for pain on the increase?

In the last five or ten years, there has been a huge promotion of pain relief as a person's right. We support that. We issue quotas for Schedule II substances, production quotas for each of the opioids. During the past eight to ten years, they have increased anywhere from four-fold to ten-fold. There's been a huge growth in the production of these products, and we've supported that. In this effort to assure adequate pain treatment, we also hope that the message gets across that these products should be treated with respect. They should not be given out lightly. There's a reason why they've been abused for centuries. We would like the medical community to recognize that all pain should not be treated with opioids, and that a patient's right to adequate pain treatment should not misconstrued as a demand for opioids. Yet, of course, when they're indicated, they should be prescribed without hesitation.

There are so many cultural, physiological, and psychological factors that go into the very personal experience of pain that trying to gauge that experience in someone else, not to mention regulate its amelioration, seems a dicey proposition to me.

I would agree with that, and from the DEA's standpoint, we aren't regulating the day-to-day decision that the doctor makes in evaluating his patient. Only the patient and the physician can do that. We ask only that when physicians approach opioids they do so with respect, that they recognize that they are brain-altering chemicals, that they be used to regulate a patient's ability to function, and that they monitor that ability. If they're drug abusers, they won't be functioning too well. If they are legitimate patients whose pain is being treated, they should improve. All the pain guidelines put out by the Federation of State Medical Boards and other bodies are moving in that direction—the monitoring of outcomes.

The physician has his work cut out for him keeping these medical, social, and regulatory issues in mind.

There are many indicators of human behavior that we're all tuned into, and the physician has to have a sense of who he or she is dealing with. I agree it can be difficult, especially in the managed-care era, where you have five or ten minutes with a patient. But the kinds of drugs we're talking about deserve the attention that the patient would need. We all have to recognize that there is a certain percentage of the population that has an addictive personality, a brain chemistry that may lend itself to more trouble than most of us might have. Physicians have to be mindful of that as they go through their day. If a doctor is not a pain specialist but just a general practitioner, and they find suddenly that everyone is coming in the door asking for a particular drug because they maybe found out it was easy to get it from them, then maybe that ought to be a signal to the doctor that they're being used as a target. Again, when opioids are necessary, medical boards and the DEA have heard the word. We've been in this arena for five or six years working very heavily with the pain-management community to make sure we all understand each other's issues, and that's been a big plus for both of us.

Peter Muryo Matthiessen, Roshi

❧

Peter Matthiessen is widely celebrated for both his fiction and his nature writing. A National Book Award winner, he has a wide-ranging vision that spans nearly half a century and covers everything from environmental and political issues to large spiritual questions. He is also a Roshi, a senior teacher of Zen. I interview him in South Florida, where he has come to participate in a writers' conference.

Would you share some thoughts about pain?

Let's talk first about pain in meditation. It's a little cliché, but in Zen practice, we say "no pain, no gain." I remember the famous teacher Yamada Roshi used to say, "Pain in the knees is the taste of *zazen*." Of course everybody—including some of the Roshis—has knee pain when they are in sitting meditation. When you sit in that position for hours you can't avoid it. In *zazenkai* retreat you may sit for as many as fourteen hours. I don't care who you are, that is very hard on the knees.

But there is a way, which I try to teach my students, of un-demonizing the pain. Pain is tremendously energizing, and when you're sitting, you are trying to empty out the upper half of your body to become just as clear as a bell or a seashell: completely clear. The energy from the pain, the heat, is all from your lower body, and you take that circle there, you take your energy from that. If you can unsubject it and simply say, "tatami mat, painting, bird song outside the window, sunlight, pain, smell of food from

the kitchen," hmm, if you can just put it there as one of the phenomena you are sensing as you sit there, it really defangs it to a
great, great degree. You're not simply saying, "pain, bad"; you are
saying "pain, green, shell, incense smell"; it just becomes part of
your surroundings. And to a great degree, by just taking away
your emotional, subjective concept of pain, you can deal with it.

Of course, there is a point where it becomes too much. Beginning meditators may even feel rage instead of going into their
sweet light. They may wait for the bell, thinking that it should
have gone off ten minutes ago, trusting their own interior clock.
We all go through that raging, but of course that raging just
makes the pain worse. Rage is all fear. If you shift your position
you just make it worse, because you can't really relieve it, so all
you do is activate it and it spreads all through your body instead
of being concentrated where you are putting your breath, in the
exhale, during the meditation. If you can focus the pain, you can
use it like a laser. You can really concentrate, really focus. So up
to a certain point, pain can be extremely useful, but there is a
point where it takes over. In my early years of Zen practice, I
would stand up and barely be able to walk after meditation. Some
people sit in a chair. I've never done that, probably mostly as a
point of vanity, but you do what you have to do. It's ridiculous
not to if you need to.

What about the pain of illness?
My wife died of cancer. She was in terrible pain a lot of the time.
I watched her undergo chemotherapy. Even though she was very
young, she was ravaged by that treatment. I wonder how well she
would have survived, even if she had come through that bout. I
told the people at the hospital that they weren't doing her any
good moving her around and weighing her and doing research on
a human body that is suffering the tortures of the damned. I told

them that I didn't want them to move her any more. I wanted them to sedate her good and plenty. Finally, when they wouldn't pay enough attention, I took her out of the hospital.

A few years ago, a friend called me up and said that another guy, a big strong fellow named John who had been on expeditions with us, had some terrible cancer and was in terrible distress in the hospital. My friend told me that John would love to hear from me. I reminded my friend that when John and I saw each other last we were in a camp up in the Northwest Territories, and we had argued. John bet me five hundred bucks I was wrong and I knew I was right and I told him, "John, I'm not going to take your bet and I'm not going to take your money." It infuriated him. He had a big ego. I asked my friend if he remembered all that and he said he did, but he still thought John would like to see me, that he had put all that away.

I didn't call right away. I looked for excuses. It was awkward. I knew what I was going to say, but I knew that *I* was going to be awkward. So I called him up and he said, "Hey, I'm in terrible shape. They're killing me with this goddamn radiation and chemo and I feel so sick all the time." He wasn't whining at all. He was telling me the facts, telling me what was being done. So he said, "You're a Zen person. Do you have any ideas about this?" I said, "John, I do. My wife died. I saw her go through a lot of bad stuff. I'm not talking to you like you're going to die; you could do a u-turn tomorrow, but let's talk about it frankly. If I were you, I would pick up and go home in the morning. For one tenth of what your family is paying for that hospitalization you can get a live-in nurse who can sedate you, medicate you any way you want, and you can live at home. You're on your farm in Vermont, your family can come see you, and if you have to die, die where you belong, at home. Don't die with a bunch of tubes in you, feeling sick to your stomach. That's no way to go."

He said, "But Jesus Christ, maybe I have a chance here in the hospital."

I answered, "Maybe you do, but what good is it going to do you? It might give you a few weeks or an extra month or two, but that's all. Is it worth it, spending your last months feeling like you do?"

He said, "I don't know if I can handle this" and he hung up. I could tell he was feeling angry. I never talked to him again, but I talked to his daughter, much later. She said, "The day after dad talked to you, he came home. We had one of the loveliest summers we ever had. We had fun, we laughed. He was at home, we had a ball, the family came and saw him in groups and so on, and he died about four or five months after you spoke to him, as well as anyone can die. Thank you very much."

When I talk to people in pain it seems to me that the pain is a dark sun. It's life but it's not life, it's pervasive, but not positive. You talked about using pain as a laser. That sounds as if you might see it as a weapon, or a tool.

That was in the context of meditation. If you're not doing meditation, where the pain can be used as a tool to coordinate with your breathing to concentrate and help you become one-pointed, to disappear into that point, and then the whole One opens up. That is the basic process of sitting meditation. You become one with your breath, breath after breath, your breath and the moment are the same, there's no future, no past, you disappear into the now, and when you do, everything opens up. That really is the first step in that enlightening experience, especially at the beginning when meditation is a new and exciting experience and miracles are popping. I've always found pain useful that way, but I've also found that it has its limit. People can take much more than they think, of course, but when they come up whining in *dokusan,*

I tell them, "Don't dismiss this until you know you can't handle any more, and I think you can handle quite a lot more." This isn't masochism at all. Everything is *upaya,* what we call skillful means. Everything is a tool, including the *zendo* itself. Even the chanting is a tool, incense is a tool, the gong, everything has been designed over centuries to enhance this feeling, even physical cleanliness, bathing before you sit. All of these things are tools, and pain is one tool among many others. So when the famous teacher Yamada Roshi said, "pain is the taste of *zazen,*" he wasn't suggesting we should all go out there and beat ourselves over the head and suffer. That wasn't his point at all.

There seems to be some innate prejudice against, discomfort with, and misapprehension of people who are in pain by people who are not. What do you think that is all about?

In both East and West, men especially are not supposed to whine about pain. We are supposed to be able to take quite a lot of it without complaint, to endure death if necessary for the common good. There's a lot of that, but more and more people are accepting the view that relieving physical pain with medication is all right. There's still a disgrace among most men about whining, but that's not entirely wrong; you don't want a nation of whiners. There is also an element of depression in physical pain. It is hard for many people to admit to depression. It is considered to be a mental illness, and any mental illness is considered disgraceful. I don't know where that comes from. Many people are depressed. I'm depressed. My whole family is full of depression, suicides, everybody. I have to face up to that. I don't try to hide it, I deal with it. Basically, I'm a very merry person. I love to horse around, even when I'm carrying bad news. But that doesn't save me from being a very depressive type any more than I might have weak eyes or a trick knee. It's part of my physical makeup, and I do believe that it is very physical, because medication alleviates it a lot. I remember one time I was driving my truck somewhere and I had a package I had just picked up from the pharmacy, and my friend, who was too snoopy by a half, grabs it and says, "Who uses this?" I told him I did and he was really startled, like he was worried that I wouldn't be easy with him, that I would start foaming at the mouth. (*laughing*)

Perhaps it's okay to expect certain things of yourself, but since somebody else's pain is something you can never fully know or understand, we have to be very compassionate with each other, especially in a health care setting, and I fear we may not always be.

I agree. There have been a number of doctors who have experimented and put themselves in as patients and been horrified at the lack of understanding and compassion, at the automatic treatment we so often get. This is not to say that there are not truly compassionate dedicated people out there, but often people are extremely callous. I remember when my wife was in Sloan Kettering, she was in a coma most of the time at the end, but sometimes when I came in, I found her agitated and upset. I knew something had happened, and it wasn't just the pain. I watched it all for a while and finally put it together that a certain nurse was involved. I was absolutely sure that this was a cold, tough little woman, brutal and automatic, who probably got a little bit of a kick out of yanking people around in bed. I felt that I had to stand up for my wife because she couldn't stand up for herself. Now I loathe the idea of falsely accusing someone. It has to be worse than anything; I just hate it. So I often bend over backwards because of that, so I asked the floor nurse where the office was and she asked me if I had a complaint and I said I was afraid I did. I told her it wasn't about her, but that I needed to speak to someone.

I finally made my way to this office, which was very well hidden, perhaps so the public couldn't easily find it, and I went in there and I said, "I'm terribly sorry, but I have to make this complaint, and even though I'm not a 100-percent sure, I think it's well founded. This is her name." The woman behind the desk sat back and very slowly smiled and said, "Thank you *very* much. We have known about this person for months. The other nurses reported it, we have seen it in the patient, but nobody from the family has come forward, which is what we needed to get her out of there. Now we have what we need."

Our health care system is driven by economics, not humanity. Sometimes the demands it makes on its workers are partly to blame. Still, in a job you do every day, a lack of compassion can easily happen if you are not vigilant.

Unless you are a rather exceptional person, the job can dehumanize you. I knew a state cop who was constantly pulling bleeding, dying people out of cars and breaking up fights and stabbings and so on. You have to be callous or you can't do that job. You have to be awfully tough. But some people can be tough-minded without losing their heart, you know. Perhaps they are the exceptional ones.

•

Pamela Bennett, R.N.

☙

Pamela Bennett is Director of Advocacy at Purdue Pharma, L.P., a leading, Connecticut-based manufacturer of opioid analgesics. I interview her at a restaurant in Palm Beach, Florida, where she is attending a conference.

It is my contention that the most interesting things about pain are the things that people don't say about it. Would you agree?

What few caregivers own up to is how important it is to be able to look at your own stuff—your sense of suffering, your fear—and embrace it. Caregivers don't want to do that. Nobody does. We do everything in our culture and our society to avoid pain, to pretend it's not there.

People who are dying have so much inside of them. They're so fearful. They're standing on a precipice looking over into the unknown, and they see muddy waters swirling beneath them and they're afraid. So often, health care professionals walk up to them and say, "Don't look over that edge. Look over there instead, at something cheerful." And yet what patients really want is someone who will come and stand next to them and say, "God, that looks pretty scary."

Do you suppose our tendency to avoid looking at things squarely in the eye is a result of associating pain with death instead of associating pain with life?

That's a very good question. Pain is a part of the life experience.

The World Health Organization looked at how well cancer pain was treated around the world, with morphine consumption being the measure. When they looked at India, they found that morphine usage was fairly low. As in many countries, there were numerous regulatory issues, but there was also another factor, namely the belief that suffering led to enlightenment, and that if you did something to hinder that suffering, you would not go on and become enlightened and fulfilled.

You're saying that morphine use was low because patients wanted to suffer?

Exactly. Pain has different meanings in different cultures. Some cultures accept the notion that God would never give you anything more than you could bear, and that to allow pain into your life is to accept a gift that shows how strong you are and how much God loves you. In other cultures, pain is a sign that you or your family members have done something wrong and you're being paid back for it. So, pain is much more than just a physiological phenomenon—it's an experience like anything else in our life.

Pain is often necessary, at least to some extent. Lepers, who have no pain, harm themselves because they can't feel pain. They look at their body as a set of appendages. In some leper colonies, a mother might tell her children to go and get the pot out of the fire, and because they don't feel any pain in their hands, the children would do so without using tongs. They would burn themselves badly, but it didn't matter because they couldn't feel it.

Pain has an important biological use. It's a warning system. Every one of us living on this earth experiences pain, whether it's physiological pain, the pain of a divorce or the pain of a love affair ending when you're sixteen. The question is, what do we do with the pain we feel? What impact does it have on us? Do we ignore it? Do we use it to reach out to someone else?

Have you come up with a paradigm for what the ideal interaction between a caregiver and a patient in pain might be?

For years I worked in a pain clinic. People who came to us had often gone to seventeen or eighteen other doctors before they came to us. They felt ignored, they felt angry, they felt sad, they felt frustrated, and they felt incredibly overwhelmed with grief and loss. Their eyes said, "You're going to tell me this is all in my head, too." They lacked touch. They lacked human interaction. One of the best things a caregiver can do is be a human being with someone else. Not just to obtain clinical information, but to really find out who that person is, to extend yourself in the interaction.

It has always been very important for me to touch my patients—whether on the shoulder or the hand—just to have some contact. Patients in pain lack that. They're vulnerable. In nursing school you are taught never to show emotion. Well you know what? Things are pretty sad sometimes, and if you're open to another person's suffering, sometimes you cry, and sometimes that's the most healing thing of all for a patient, to see that their caregiver cares.

Showing emotion is showing compassion. Shouldn't that be the obvious core of any caregiving interaction?

It should be, but it isn't, and that goes back to people having a lack of compassion for themselves. If we're not willing to accept ourselves, with our own frailties and humanities, how can we embrace someone else? Caregivers who feel that they have to be perfect—to know all the answers within the 3.5 minutes that they're allotted to see a patient—become machines. They lose the ability to feel compassion. They expect the patient to function under duress because that is how they have to function.

You mentioned that in nursing school you were taught not to show emo-

tion. *Do you suppose that such instruction in dispassion had as its goal greater professional competence?*

To some extent, yes. One has to be able to function in the moment with clear clinical judgment. But we're all human. We can't be machines. Health care can be sad sometimes. How can you not be moved as you watch a fifteen-year-old girl die, a fifteen-year-old girl who couldn't even finish a sentence when you first met her because she was in so much pain, but who, with proper pain control, was able to record a song that was played at her own funeral?

Do any other particularly moving stories come to mind from your advocacy work?

I've always been a fighter for the underserved. To me, everyone in health care should be a patient advocate. That's why we're there doing what we're doing. If it isn't, why are we there? Surely not for money or glory. It should be because we care about people. I remember some hearings about the intractable pain law in the state of Colorado. I listened to the deans of the medical school and the nursing school and the pharmacy school talk about the good things they were doing in pain management. They had made some strides, but frankly were not nearly where they needed to be. Then I heard one gentleman talk about what great care they gave their patients at an HMO. As it happened, I had spent the previous two weeks trying to get that very HMO to pay for generic morphine for a woman, a single parent with breast cancer. They were denying her because they said they had a lifetime maximum on pain treatment. What kind of great care was that?

I sent a note about my experience up to the senator conducting the hearings, and he asked me to testify the following week. I told him I was just a nurse, not a professor. I didn't have lots of letters after my name. Nobody would listen to me. His answer was, "If you don't speak up, who will? How will we know what's going on at the bedside if you don't tell us?" That was a powerful lesson to me in overcoming my sense of inadequacy and doing what was right for all patients under my care.

It seems unconscionable and inconceivable that there could possibly be a lifetime maximum on pain control.

Every insurance company has different benefits they will pay for. Often these details are hidden amidst reams of pages. Unless you're in pain, unless you are suffering from some catastrophic and painful illness, you're not likely to look and see what your pain benefit is. Can you imagine the effect that a spending limit had on the woman I mentioned, a woman who had metastatic disease eating at her flesh, bones, and nerves, creating unimaginable agony? The HMO said, "Sorry, we'll only spend this much money on you." How was that woman going to care for her children? What were they going to have to watch her endure? What would that put into their hearts and minds for the rest of their lives? What does that say about us as a culture? What does it say about us as human beings?

Wouldn't somebody in that position go into hospice? Doesn't hospice carry a whole different set of benefits?

You have to know about hospice. If you ask most hospice providers, they will tell you that the length of stay in hospice is very short because people come to it late. Oftentimes people aren't even informed that hospice is an option until just before they die. So yes, that's an option, but you have to meet the criteria for it, and you have to know it's there.

Earlier you said that people in pain just want their caregiver to listen. Could you expand on that?

Pain is a universal experience, and an opportunity for us to show compassion to one another. Compassion, which I'm sorry to say is largely lacking in society, means being willing to step outside yourself. It's an issue that transcends health care. How many people, for example, have had a family tragedy? How many children have had to deal with a bullet? You can look at almost any situation in life and ask if you're going to walk in fear or walk in love. To understand someone in pain, you have to listen. Chronic pain patients want people to listen to them, but so do people who are not in pain. Everybody feels that they need people to listen better, to understand them better. Everybody.

Are there studies showing whether acting in a compassionate way increases the efficacy of medications or procedures?

Let me answer your question by telling you about John. John was a forty-year-old gentleman who never drank, cussed, smoked and didn't go out with women who did. He ate tofu and he jogged five miles a day. He did everything right in his life, and he ended up with the most aggressive form of lung cancer I've ever seen. He had metastases everywhere. He came to a pain center in Boston where I was working. One doctor had given him an intrathecal pump—that's an implanted device that delivers pain medication directly to the spinal fluid, and quit treating him the next day. Another doctor had given him an epidural catheter, another form of spinal cord pain control, but wouldn't push the dose enough to make John comfortable.

John came to us in the company of his wife. His pain was nine on a scale of one to ten. He could barely get out of the chair. His anxiety level was sky-high. He was totally climbing out of his skin. After about a week and a half, we got his pain under control and then set our sights on his anxiety. He was terrified the pain would come back, because that had been his experience for so long. When we accomplished that, we asked what we could do for him next. He said, "Pamela, I'd like you to get me a double hospital bed. There's nothing I like better than sleeping with my wife, and I can't do that in this bed I have now." I was never able to do that for him, by the way.

Two months before he died, John suffered bilateral iatrogenic hip fractures. The radiation he received had so weakened his bones that the weight of his body broke them. I went to his room and asked him if he wanted a back rub. He said, "Oh yeah!" Now, it wasn't that I gave great backrubs, but this guy rolled over on his fractured hips so I would rub his back. That's how much people need contact. That's how much people need connection.

A month before he died, John became a paraplegic because of a tumor in his spinal cord. His pain had been well managed for weeks, but all of a sudden it was out of control again, and he became very anxious. The hospital psychologist was with me that day, and although she had always wanted to talk to him and let him know her services were available, John wasn't interested. Later that day I got a call saying that John was asking for the psychologist. She had left, but I had her paged and she came back to the hospital. I figured if he was asking for her, something was up. I went up to John's room to wait for the psychologist and he asked me for a hand rub. I was sitting there rubbing his hand and he said, "Pamela, I think I'm going to die tonight. I don't know what to do. Do you think I should talk to my family about it?" I asked him if he had ever talked to his family about death before and he said, "No, we're always talking about how I'm going to beat this thing and how I'm going to live." I told him I didn't think it was wrong to tell the truth.

The psychologist came and we talked for a while, and then John's wife and kids showed up. The kids were more interested in the television. The wife was loving and affectionate. The kids were hungry, and I took them down to the cafeteria and then to watch *The Simpsons* on TV in the lounge so John could be alone with his wife and the psychologist. *The Simpsons* episode was about a guy who died in the hospital. The kids were glued to the TV, and I was thinking that in a few minutes I'm going to have to take them up to their father's room and he's going to tell them he's going to die. It was unbelievable.

When we finally did go up, John was in tears and asked his kids to sit on the bed with him. Then he said, "Children, I think I'm going to die tonight." As soon as he said it, this whole wave came out of him. The relief was amazing. The kids screamed. Two of them almost threw up, everyone just lost it. After a minute, John told me he wanted to go home. That took a little doing, but I arranged it, got his discharge meds, talked to hospice. I was intent on it. The janitor actually helped us wheel John's bed to the car. It turned out that he was the one who had been the most compassionate of all.

The janitor.

That's right. He'd been coming in to see John every night. He'd brought pictures of his family to show John, they had talked about fatherhood. It was hard not to contrast that with caregivers at rounds talking about this or that diagnosis but never really recognizing John's individuality. Anyway, we took John home. A neighbor went and filled his prescription. As soon as he was home he was a different person. His pain was so tied up with his anxiety and his spiritual issues. He looked at his daughter and he said, "I hear you made a pie. I want a big piece." He hadn't eaten in days! He sat down at the kitchen table. We all laughed. He said, "Now I feel like a bowel movement." He'd been constipated for days. Suddenly he could just let everything go.

Did John die that night?

He ended up living another month, at home, in his garden, with his family. Everyone got to be with one another, to say the things they needed to say. And, to finally answer your question about the role of compassion in pain management, his dose of pain medication actually decreased during that time.

Rabbi Rami Shapiro

 especialista

Rabbi Rami Shapiro is a specialist in interfaith issues, a noted lecturer, and the author of several acclaimed spiritual books. I interview him at his temple in South Miami–Dade County, Florida, a couple of weeks before he is due to move to Los Angeles to take over the directorship of Metivta, an organization that helps train rabbis in meditative practice.

I'm sure you have seen quite a few people in deep pain in your years as a congregation rabbi.

Maybe the fundamental question is, Why is it not okay for people to be happy? Maybe the question is, What should people be? If the answer is that they should be happy, then what is wrong with going after happiness? What was wrong with peace and love in the 1960s? Why are there only certain legitimate avenues for happiness as opposed to other ways that are culturally determined to be not legitimate? I don't know the answer, but I would suspect that for all of our seeming desire for happiness, the culture doesn't really want us to be. The culture has a different ideal in mind. If you look at Western culture, our ideal person would be Jesus. The whole point of being Jesus was to be crucified. And so this whole notion of carrying our cross, and ultimately being crucified on it as the means to redemption and salvation, is systemic to at least Western culture. I don't know what we would say about the East. I could speculate. But certainly in the West, in countries where the culture is rich in Christian heritage, in Christian tradition, there has got to be some powerful, if deeply sublimated notion that we're all supposed to suffer. If we don't suffer, something is wrong with us. If that's true, then you can take a look at our attitudes toward all kinds of behaviors and activities and substances that can reduce if not remove suffering and say well, those aren't really allowed, or they're just allowed in small amounts, so as to not get us away from the fundamental point of our existence, which is to suffer.

There is a parallel on the Eastern side. Let's take Buddhism as the dominant tradition there. The Buddha said that his whole teaching is about suffering and the ending of suffering. I'm speculating here, but I wonder if that is very different from the Western notion of suffering and the salvation that comes through suffering. In Buddhism, there is no salvation through suffering. You want to end suffering. You end suffering by ending desire. In the West, suffering and desire are not necessarily equated. You aren't really allowed to end suffering.

That brings us to this whole notion of pain and pain management and all of that. There has got to be something intrinsic, hidden very deep in our Western psyche, that allows us to say patently absurd statements such as, "We can't give this person morphine in the dosage that she needs to eliminate or minimize the pain that she's in—even though her life expectancy is six to eight weeks— because she'll become an addict." That's an absurd statement, but we say it, and we don't think it's absurd. We say it and then we justify it somehow. But underneath the justification there has to be some other paradigm that we've all accepted that says, "Well, that makes sense. We wouldn't want this person to become an addict." Even though they're not going to live out the next six months. So that is something we need to explore, uncover, and take a look at to see if it's really a rational paradigm to be following.

The other thing is that whole Calvinist approach to life. John Calvin said that our lives are predestined, that we are predestined to be saved or not to be saved. I'm not Christian, but I don't think even Christians take this literally anymore. Still, the notion is that whatever happens to us is supposed to happen to us. Since you can't know whether you're saved or not, the Calvinist doctrine was that you looked for symptoms of salvation. A symptom of salvation is being successful—working hard and making money and living the good life, whatever the good life back then was. I think that's also part of the Western, specifically the American psyche—that hard work and perseverence are going to pay off. Or they should pay off. That's our fundamental truth there. That means that suffering is part of it. We put in a lot of hard work, go through the school of hard knocks, that there is something to be learned, and gained, through suffering. And I'm sure there is, to some extent. The question would be, Is suffering the only place we learn? Can we say, I've got the lesson, let's turn the suffering off?

A number of women in our congregation are suffering from advanced breast cancer. One woman in particular said to me that she was at some meeting and someone was talking to her about the lessons that she learns, that her soul needed to learn, from this turn of life. She said, "I've learned as much as I want to learn. Let's graduate this class. I don't need this anymore." But whether we're talking religious, or we're talking New Age or the kind of thinking you find on "Oprah," there's always a purpose and a meaning to our suffering, which means that ending it is somehow counter to what needs to be done. So we are all willing to accept suffering because somehow we are going to benefit from it. Either it's salvation through pain or it's the soul's lesson or something like that.

It strikes me that when we go to a health care practitioner in pursuit of amelioration of pain, we are putting ourselves in their hands in a simi-

lar way to the way in which a congregant puts himself in your hands. There seems to be a parallel between being a priest or a rabbi and being a physician in the religion called "Science." I know that that there is an abdication of personal responsibility that happens when we go to the doctor, and that some of us take great comfort in handing over the reigns. Yet, at the same time, that trust, appropriate or not, may be violated when suffering is not reduced or eliminated—when what we are surrendering for is not given.

There's an upside to that kind of surrender of responsibility, and there's a limit to it. I have no problem surrendering my self-reliance when it comes to experts in things that are way over my head. I had to go the other day for a high-tech medical test. You know, I'm not going to take the time to become a technician, or build the machine and do it to myself. I'm going to rely on all these people and assume that they know what they're doing. At the same time, we have to realize that we are placing our trust in the hands of someone who is limited by a paradigm—by their own model. If I go to a physician and I'm hoping to alleviate pain, and the physician can only go so far because of his or her philosophy of medicine, there's a limit to what that person can do. It's good on the one hand, because I don't need to become an M.D. to figure out what I need to do, but there's a limit to it because the M.D. I go to can only go as far as her training and ability allow.

In religion, it's the same thing. Someone comes to me hoping to alleviate some spiritual pain they're having. They believe that God is angry with them. I deal with a lot of people who come in believing that God is punishing them. My own personal philosophy doesn't allow for that. God isn't a self-conscious being who knows who I am. My theology is very different. So the "cure" I can offer them is a spiritual practice, a contemplative meditative practice, that ultimately gets them beyond the whole notion of the duality of themselves and God and the whole notion of punishment—maybe pushing the envelope of Judaism. But that's not what they want.

What a more conventional clergy-person would never do is to say, "You know what you need? You need Jesus! You need to become a Christian and you'll feel much better." They're not going to do that. They're only going to take you as far as their system allows. I guess that's the point I was making with medicine as well. There's a system, and the person that you're dealing with can only go within that system. So whether it's clergy or scientists or M.D.s or whatever it is, they're all working within a specific system. And it's true with your alternative therapies as well. I know chiropractors who believe that chiropractic will cure everything. Once I even saw a serious film, not "Saturday Night Live," where the implication was that had Hitler had his spine adjusted early on, we never would have had World War II and the Holocaust! People sometimes forget that systems have their limits.

The last thing I want to say about surrender regards the whole notion that we should be self-reliant. That also feeds into the maintaining the pain thing. I should be happy. I should be able to make myself happy without reliance on other people or on medication. I should be able to go through whatever life throws at me without being rocked by it. That's sort of the ideal we set for ourselves. But that's an incredible thing to think—that we should be able to do this. When you realize that we cannot, that human beings were not created that way, that we really do suffer and feel pain, that some of it is simply a chemical imbalance, you have this incredible question: I'm bipolar II, I'm manic-depressive, is there something spiritually important about that? Did my soul choose depression so that it could experience those things that it needs to experience and move on in its evolution?

That is a wonderful metaphysical way of excusing a physical ailment that is easily fixed. If you can take someone who is manic-depressive and successfully medicate them—not so that they are smiling like the village idiot but so they are no longer manic depressive and are satisfied and basically happy people going through life without such highs and lows—what's wrong with that? It's all jars and pills—all chemicals. Why is it that one set of chemicals, the set that causes pain, that the body generates on its own, is more sacred, more holy, more valid, than another set of chemicals that we can introduce into the body that removes that pain? This whole notion that toughing it out and being self-reliant is better than being a weak character and surrendering to some biochemistry that might alleviate pain is a difficult one. I don't think we've really dealt with those issues.

The self-reliance issue evokes a separation between doctor and patient that echoes the religious duality of Christian thinking—the notion of God being distinct from man. Moreover, self-reliance implies a lack of connection between people, between patient and caregiver, for example. That lack of empathy, that notion of us and them, makes it a lot easier to leave someone in pain, harder to ask for relief, and makes proper pain management difficult.

That's a very interesting point to make. Certainly in conventional religious thought there is duality between Creation and God, Nature and God, human beings and God, human beings and Nature. There are all these splits—all these divisions. That's just theological talk. In reality there are none of those divisions. In mystical teachings, whether Eastern or Western, Jewish, Christian, Hindu, Buddhist, Muslim, Sufi, whatever, it all comes down to the fact that everything is one. But when you go into a setting like a doctor's office, there are all kinds of very clear messages that here is the high priest and you are the supplicant. Some of that is necessary and some of that is unnecessary. Some of it is driven by a need for me, the patient, to feel comfortable going to the priest/doctor, but a lot of it is driven by the economics of the profession.

I have a psychotherapist friend who sits with her people for the fifty-minute hour, and then when the fifty minutes is up, just keeps going. She doesn't get extra pay for it, she just gets so involved in the lives of these people, they're so interesting to her, she becomes so empathic to them, that if she has an extra half-hour or hour, she'll just give them two hours without economic incentive. Many other therapists will stop right when the time is up, even if the patient is in the middle of some incredibly devastating thing. When I go to the doctor there are a million people waiting behind me; I've got my eight or ten minutes, and no more.

That's the economic reality of the situation; the doctor doesn't have time to be empathetic. But there's a certain usefulness in that distance. It can make the job easier. There's a need to disassociate from other people's pain. We can know that so and so is hurting, but it doesn't really impact on us. Not because we're heartless and cruel, but because if all that pain did impact on us, we couldn't function. So we begin to build these defenses against it. Maybe that's how you allow some of these chronic pain conditions to continue even though you know there's a remedy for it, and you don't do anything actively to advocate for changing of the law or the system. We can abstract ourselves to some extent. We can go home, and we can say, "Well that was work, and this is my life. It's different."

One would hope that the choice of a health care career is based more on compassion than it is on prestige and economics. Can you think of any particular examples of separateness or compassion?

I've been in situations where stillborn babies were delivered, bagged, and sent to the morgue, and no one ever saw them. One time, however, we knew the baby was going to be born deceased, and the hospital had made arrangements for the birth to take place in a private room. The baby was swaddled and brought to them, and they were left with the baby for as long as they needed to make that connection. I was with them, the nurses were there, the doctors were there. It was just human beings at their compassionate best.

Then I've seen situations where someone dies and before you can say good-bye the sheet has been thrown over them and the bed is being wheeled out so as to free the room for someone else. It goes both ways. I think you're right. People who go into the helping professions do intend to go in as helpers, but our caregivers—nurses, doctors, therapists, hospice workers—are so overworked, so stressed, stretched so thin, and are given so little support in dealing with other people's suffering as well as their own, that they just can't do what the individual client or patient would want them to do. They don't have the time, the energy, the expertise or the internal support system to pull it off.

What have we left out?

The Book of Job. The whole story of Job was about this incredibly successful person who, on a bet, God basically destroys. He kills off his kids, kills off his business, reduces him from a healthy person to a very, very sick individual under extraordinary pain, mental and physical, just to see what happens, to see if he'll maintain his loyalty to God or not. He does, in a sense. He holds out to the end. He refuses to accept any responsibility for what has happened to him. He knows he's innocent of any crime. The whole karmic thing is not acceptable to Job. Job says to God, "Tell me what's going on!" God shows up and says to Job, "There's no way you can understand what's going on in the universe. There is no philosophy or paradigm that's going to make sense of it for you. There's just this completely wild, overflowing energy that I generate." And then Job goes "I get it." He has an enlightenment experience. The best translation of this, from a Zen perspective, is by Stephen Mitchell. Job has an awakening. The story concludes with Job getting his kids back, all new kids, by the way, not the old kids, but he gets a whole new life.

So, in the West, we talk about the patience of Job. The story itself doesn't suggest that Job is patient. Job is very demanding. Job wants to know why there is suffering in the world. But we took that story, which could be very, very existentially liberating, and we turned it into a very safe story. Nice Job. He sits there and he takes it and he takes it and he takes it, abuse upon abuse upon abuse. Isn't that wonderful? His patience is what carries him through. It's not! It's his perseverance to know why God does this. We can't deal with that as a culture, so we make it patience. We make it "You have the patience of Job. Ultimately, God will reward you." That's the hidden message, not of the Bible story itself, but of the way we have taken the Bible story. The story itself is much more radical. We need to think about it.

Toward Compassionate Pain Management

When I was a little boy, my father made frequent late-night housecalls. I know, because I was a light sleeper, and he always woke me when he left. Although his career later took on media, professorial, administrative, and literary dimensions, there is no doubt in my mind that he chose the path of a physician because he wanted to help people. His example taught me that physicians must first and foremost be healers, that the respect and the remuneration that come with the job should be secondary goals if they are goals at all, and that they should flow as the result of compassionate action. I believe we have lost sight of this, both in defining the roles of physicians and in structuring and executing the delivery of health care. The practice of medicine has become tech-heavy. Many cutting-edge therapies are specialized procedures requiring doctors to emphasize technical aspects at the expense of relationships with patients. This is not the fault of the physicians themselves, but of the economics behind the system.

The more mechanical the practice of medicine, the more easily it becomes a business lacking in human warmth and compassion.

Also, the sheer volume of information that underpins modern medicine—and I include here effective alternative modalities such as acupuncture, herbology, energy therapies, and the like—continues to increase at an exponential rate. This puts a tremendous burden on physicians, who must work impossible hours if they are to stay up to date, particularly when regulation and managed care are thrown into the mix. The physician is between a rock and a hard place, with a society crying out for a level of care that most physicians want desperately to provide but often find they cannot. This is nowhere more evident than in the treatment of chronic pain.

Pain clinics help. Springing up all over the country, they feature teams of caregivers providing everything from physical therapy and palliative medications and procedures to counseling for the loneliness, anxiety, and depression that so often accompany chronic pain. Chronic pain patients must take, and be given, more responsibility for managing that pain. Empowering the patient is critical, because empowerment means a positive attitude, and a positive attitude provides relief, distraction, and a rich soil for the roots of healing. Grassroots bills of rights for patients are important in redefining the contract between physician and patient, but physicians must be open to this partnership, too. According to many of them, medical students grow less compassionate and more cynical as their training proceeds, and course work in medical ethics—which deals primarily with theories and facts as opposed to human tendencies and feelings—may do little to stanch the leak. It would be convenient if there were some way to screen for compassion in medical school admissions, but this would fail to take into account the fact that compassion often develops through experience and over time. All the same, we must never forget that medical competence and compassion are two wings of the same bird. Without either, a caregiver is unable to fly.

If the doctor/patient relationship is to become a true partnership, the patient must accept it, too. If doctors have too much power, it is because we have all willingly given it. Physicians must remember that theirs is a service profession, and patients must not sit idly back and wait for miracles. They must no longer fear their physicians, no longer see them as adversaries, no longer feel that their physicians have more power over their plight than they do themselves. They must listen, ask questions and learn. As the science and technology of medicine evolve, conditions that were previously dismissed are suddenly revealed to be genuine, and the organic basis for seemingly undocumentable pain is often discovered. This underscores the fact that physicians must always give patients the benefit of the doubt.

The business of managing chronic pain is one of the fastest-growing areas in medicine, and one that is receiving a bloom of public interest. Business does not tend to be compassionate, so compassion must be mandated. The new JCAHO rules establishing pain as a fifth vital sign and dictating that a person's pain be taken seriously, properly evaluated, promptly treated, regularly reassessed, and that the patient be referred to a pain specialist if need be are a start, but do not take into account the fact that no matter how many measuring scales and tables are employed, pain is not just an objective condition, but a symbol of a subjective suffering.

Pain relief must become a primary moral imperative of the practice of medicine, but while the reality is that someone has to pay for pain management, on so many levels not treating chronic pain *costs far more than treating it*. An acute-care model—that is, waiting for things to become truly debilitating—costs far more than early and aggressive treatment. The financial burden of chronic pain in lost wages, lost productivity, lost time, may amount to as much as $100 billion a year. Psychotherapy, exercise, relaxation techniques, and alternative therapies are far less costly than high-tech scans and complex surgical procedures, and the early and appropriate use of pain relievers short-circuits the destructive cycle of chronic pain, saving dollars and heartache at the same time. In a future model, all medical specialties must be made more aware of the human, medical, and financial costs of chronic pain, and the artificial division of mind and body must be relinquished so that the patient is always treated as a person.

The media have become the judge, jury, and executioner in our culture, and news stories about the abuse of pain medications by addicts abound. These articles usually sensationalize addiction while conveniently ignoring the harsh reality of the chronic pain patient who uses opioid analgesics for a legitimate medical purpose. They take doctors to task for doing what they literally *vowed* to do, namely to eliminate human suffering. Sensationalizing violent drug-related crimes and overdoses serves the news organs far more than the public, and whips up support for an expensive and ineffective war on drugs that fails to reduce either the product, through successful interdiction, or the demand, through education and social programs.

Chronic pain patients are perhaps the most unfortunate victims of the war on drugs. For political reasons, they suddenly have to fear that their lifeline will be cut, or that they will become the objects of suspicion and derision. The fact is that in all but a minuscule number of cases, chronic pain patients have nothing to do with either abusing pharmaceuticals or profiting from them. Study after study shows that people in chronic pain don't get high from opioid analgesics, they get relief; and while they may require assistance in frequency and dosing, they are medication users, not drug abusers. Criminals who use and sell drugs, and pain patients depending on prescription medications to live a normal life, *have no intersection whatsoever*.

Some people claim that people in pain are not disabled. They are mistaken. Chronic pain patients suffer poor attention, brain hormone abnormalities, fatigue, mood disorders, and impaired mental and physical performance. Like many other disabled people they need advocacy, but unlike many other disabled people they cannot be their own advocates. For the most part, they don't have the required stamina or clarity of mind because they are too busy dealing with their pain. We must strive to validate their experience rather than judge it, for validation eases emotional pain in the same way that medications ease physical pain.

Our culture turns away from people in pain because they remind us that what has happened to them may some day happen to us, and that all of us are going to die. Can we eliminate all pain? No. Can we control our prejudices and attitudes and actions? Yes. Compassion is at the heart of that control. Compassion is not just a warm-and-fuzzy term, it is a tremendous social, spiritual, and economic force. Instead of turning *away* from the needy, we must turn *toward* them with compassion. In doing so, we assure ourselves the powerful positive results, both psychic and physical, that compassion brings.

Resource Guide

American Academy of Craniofacial Pain
516 W. Pipeline Road
Hurst, Texas 76053
Phone: 817/282-1501
Fax: 817/282-8012
E-mail: central@aahnfp.org
http://www.aahnfp.org

American Academy of Pain Management
13947 Mono Way #A
Sonora, CA 95370
Phone: 209/533-9744
Fax: 209/533-9750
www.aapainmanage.org

American Academy of Pain Medicine
4700 W. Lake
Glenview, IL 60025
Phone: 847/375-4731
Fax: 847/375-6331
E-mail: aapm@amctec.com
www.painmed.org

American Academy of Physical Medicine and Rehabilitation
One IBM Plaza, Suite 2500
Chicago, IL 60611–3604
Phone: 312/464-9700
Fax: 312/464-0227
E-mail: info@aapmr.org
http://www.aapmr.org

American Alliance of Cancer Pain Initiatives
1300 University Ave., Rm. 4720
Madison, WI 53706
Phone: 608/265-4013
Fax: 608/265-4014
http://www.aacpi.org/home.html

American Association of Osteopathic Pain Management & Sclerotherapy, Inc.
303 S. Ingram Court
Middleton, DE 19707
Phone: 302/376-8080

American Association of Nurse Anesthetists
222 S. Prospect Avenue
Park Ridge, IL 60068
Phone: 847/692-7050
http://www.aana.com

American Chronic Pain Association (ACPA)
P.O. Box 850
Rocklin, CA 95677
Phone: 810/533-3231
Fax: 916/632-3208
E-mail: ACPA@pacbell.net
www.theacpa.org

American Council for Headache Education
19 Mantua Road
Mt. Royal, NJ 08061
Phone: 856/423-0258
Fax: 856/423-0082
E-mail: achehq@talley.com
www.achenet.com

American Pain Foundation
201 N. Charles Street, Suite 710
Baltimore, MD 21201-4111
Phone: 888/615-PAIN (7246)
http://www.painfoundation.org

American Society of Clinical Oncology
1900 Duke Street, Suite 200
Alexandria, VA 22314
Phone: 703/299-0150
Fax: 703/299-1044
E-mail: asco@asco.org
http://www.asco.org

American Society of Regional Anesthesia and Pain Medicine
P.O. Box 11086
Richmond, VA 23230–1086
Phone: 804/282-0010
Fax: 804/282-0090
E-mail: asra@societyhq.com
http://www.asra.com

Anesthesia Patient Safety Foundation (APSF)
4246 Colonial Park Drive
Pittsburgh, PA 15227–2621
Phone: 412/882-8040
E-mail: info@apsf.org
http://www.apsf.org

City of Hope Pain/Palliative Care Resource Center
National Medical Center
Department of Nursing Research & Education
1500 East Duarte Road
Duarte, CA 91010
Fax: c/o Stacey Pejsa, Pain Resource Coordinator, at 626/301-8941
http://www.cityofhope.org

International Association for the Study of Pain
IASP Secretariat
909 NE 43rd St., Suite 306
Seattle, WA 98105–6020
Phone: 206/547-6409
Fax: 206/547-1703
E-mail: IASP@locke.hs.washington.edu
http://www.iasp.org

National Chronic Pain Outreach Association (NCPOA)
7979 Old Georgetown Rd., Suite 100
Bethesda, MD 20814–2429
Phone: 301/652-4948
Fax: 301/907-0745

National Committee on the Treatment of Intractable Pain (NCTIP)
c/o Wayne Coy, Jr.
Cohn and Marks
1920 N St. NW, Ste. 300
Washington, D.C. 20036
Phone: 202/452-4836
Fax: 202/293-4827

National Headache Foundation (NHF)
428 W. Saint James Pl., 2nd fl.
Chicago, IL 60614-2750
Phone: 773/388-6399;
888/NHF-5552
Fax: 773/525-7357
E-mail: info@headaches.org
www.headaches.org

Oncolink,University of Pennsylvania Cancer Center
3400 Spruce St.—2 Donner
Philadelphia, PA 19104-4283
Fax: 215/349-5445
http://www.cancer.med.upenn.edu

Pain & Policy Studies Group
406 Science Drive, Suite 202
Madison, WI 53711-1068
Phone: 608/263-7662
E-mail: ppsq@med.wisc.edu
http://www.medsch.wisc.edu/painpolicy/

Pain Research Group
1100 Holcombe, Box 221
Houston, TX 77030
Phone: 713/745-3470

Fax: 713/745-3475
http://prg.mdanderson.org

Peaceful Dwelling
33 Chapel Ave.
Brookhaven, NY 11719-9401
Phone: 631/776-2444
Fax: 631/776-2442
E-mail: info@peacefuldwelling.org

Puzzle of Pain
http://www.oregonlive.com/special/series/old/pain.ssf

The Vulvar Pain Foundation
203 1/2 North Main St., Suite 203
Graham, NC 27253
Phone: 336/226-0704
Fax: 336/226-8518
http://www.vulvarpainfoundation.org

The University of Texas M.D. Anderson Cancer Center
1515 Holcombe Blvd.
Houston, TX 77030
Phone: 800/392-1611, 713/792-6161
http://www.mdanderson.org

American Pain Society
4700 W. Lake Ave.
Glenview, IL 60025
Phone: 847/375-4715
Fax: 877/734-8758 [toll free]
E-mail: info@ampainsoc.org
www.ampainsoc.org

American Pain Society Branches:

Southern Pain Society
4700 W. Lake Avenue
Glenview, IL 60025
Phone: 847/375-4700

Fax: 847/375-4792
E-mail: jkokkines@amctec.com

Eastern Pain Association
P.O. Box 11086
Richmond, VA 23230–1086
Phone: 804/282-0063
Fax: 804/282-0090
E-mail: kay@societyhq.com

Greater Philadelphia Pain Society
Park Towne Place, Suite 108 North
2200 Ben Franklin Parkway
Philadelphia, PA 19130
Phone: 215/557-9705
Fax: 215/557-9683

Midwest Pain Society
4700 W. Lake Avenue
Glenview, IL 60025
Phone: 847/375-4730
Fax: 847/375-4777
E-mail: jkokkines@amctec.com

New England Pain Association
1910 Byrd Avenue, Suite 100
Richmond, VA 23230–1086
Phone: 804/282-4011
Fax: 804/282-0090

Western USA Pain Society
8700 Beverly Blvd.
Los Angeles, CA 90048
Phone: 310/855-8030 ext.314
Fax: 310/659-3928

Glossary

anxiolytics. drugs that counter anxiety

arachnoid cyst. a cyst in the delicate membrane that encloses the brain and spinal cord

arachnoiditis. inflammation of the delicate membrane that encloses the brain and spinal cord

arteriovenous malformation. a congenital lesion that opens an artery into a vein

biofeedback. a technique for making unconscious or involuntary bodily functions perceptible in order to consciously affect them

bodhisattva. a Buddhist term for someone who is worshipped because they refrain from entering nirvana in order to save others

botulinum toxin. the virulent product of the bacteria Clostridium botulinum

chakra. a term in yoga, ayurvedic medicine, and New Age parlance that refers to any of several points of physical or spiritual energy in the human body

Descartes, René. the seventeenth-century French philosopher and mathematician best known for the phrase "I think, therefore I am"

dokusan. Japanese term for a personal interview between teacher and student

endogenous. caused by factors inside the organism or system

facet hypertrophy. overgrowth of small, smooth surface of bone

fascia. a fibrous membrane covering, supporting, and separating muscles

fibromyalgia. a group of nonspecific illnesses characterized by pain, joint stiffness, fatigue, insomnia, and more.

healing touch. an energy-based approach to healing mind and body using principles dating back 5,000 years

herniation. development of a protrusion or projection of an organ through the cavity that normally contains it

hyperalgesia. excessive sensitivity to pain

hyperesthesia. increased sensitivity to sensory input

hypertension. high blood pressure

hyperthyroidism. a condition caused by excessive secretions of the thyroid gland

iatrogenic. a disorder caused by treatment

intrathecal. referring to the space under the arachnoid membrane of the brain or spinal cord

Kubler-Ross. Dr. Elisabeth Kubler-Ross. A Swiss-American physician noted for her work on death and dying

limbic System. a group of brain structures, including the hippocampus, amygdala, and more, that is associated with motivated behaviors and arousal, and stimulates the endocrine system and the autonomic nervous system

Marfan's syndrome. a hereditary condition of connective tissue, bones, muscles, and ligaments

MCAT. Medical College Admission Test

metastatic. usually a cancer that has spread from the original site to multiple locations

methadone. a synthetic analgesic drug often used in treating addiction to more dangerous narcotics

migraines. paroxysmal attacks of headache, often associated with light sensitivity, nausea, and more

myofascia. a muscle and its associated connective tissue

myositis. inflammation of muscle tissue

nociception. brain's perception of pain

Noloxone. a drug that has no analgesic effect, primarily used to treat overdose and in research

opioid analgesic. a class of synthetic pain medications related to, but not derived from opium

palliative. functioning to relieve or alleviate but not cure

polymyalgia. a poorly understood condition marked by muscle pain, most common in women and the elderly

psychosomatic. concerning the relationship between mind and body

sansei. Japanese term for a son or daughter of first generation Japanese parents who is born and educated in the United States

Schedule II. a federal regulation requiring that the prescription and distribution of a certain class of medications, including opioid analgesics, be controlled by law

sciatica. severe pain along the course of the sciatic nerve, in the leg

spinal stenosis. a narrowing of the spinal canal

Selective Serotonin Reuptake Inhibitor (SSRI). a member of a class of compounds that modulate mood and brain function by affecting the metabolism of the neurotransmitter serotonin

suboccipital neuralgia. a sharp pain below the back part of the skull

thalamic. pertaining to the thalamus

thalamus. the part of the brain that receives all sensory information, other than olfaction, and relays the information onward

transcutaneous electrical stimulator. a device that applies an electrical current through the skin to an affected part

trigeminal neuralgia. a sharp pain along the course of the trigeminal nerve, also known as facial neuralgia

upaya. Japanese term for skillful means

varicosity. a state of abnormal swelling or dilation

zazen. Japanese term for seated meditation

zazenkai. Japanese term for a one-day meditation retreat

zendo. Japanese term for a place for Zen meditation